T0386416

"Melissa has fearlessly taken a topic of paramount importance and boldly deconstructs the complex concepts of sexuality and body image through her personally unique and radical lens. Fabello, in an effort to share this essential knowledge discovered through her dissertation—a subject that she readily acknowledges is inaccessible outside of the exclusionary work within academia—has managed to translate her findings into a book where the information is both authentically and accessibly shared; allowing the world to learn about critical subjects like 'skin hunger,' 'sensuality', and 'intimacy' (to name a just a few) in a way that feels both approachable and profoundly personal. *Appetite* is authentic, relatable, flawlessly researched, and sprinkled with humor; a combination that makes it an imperative read. This book is not only comprehensive and inclusive but the depth (and breadth) of her findings are astoundingly masterful. Whether you are a practitioner, educator, researcher, advocate or someone who simply wants to learn more and experience the most amazing braingasm of your life... *Appetite* is for you."

– **Jes Baker,** Author of *Things No One Will Tell Fat Girls: A Handbook for Unapologetic Living*

"Melissa Fabello is a rare voice of reason in our weight-obsessed, food-phobic society. With nuance and clarity, she unpacks the lies and half-truths we've been told about food, bodies, and sexuality, and offers a much-needed intersectional-feminist perspective on these topics—while also managing to be incredibly fun to read. Her work has helped inform and deepen my thinking on disordered eating and social justice, and I'm so grateful to have her as a colleague in the fight to dismantle diet culture."

– **Christy Harrison**, Author of *Anti-Diet: Reclaim Your Time, Money, Wellbeing, and Happiness Through Intuitive Eating*

"Melissa's approach on addressing skin hunger and anorexia illustrates the complexities and nuances of eating disorders. It reminds us that while eating disorders are often a disconnect from self and others, people suffering still have desires for connection. It reminds me as a clinician to hold the various nuances of eating disorders as I work with people suffering from them. And it gives hope that a light of recovery remains in people even in the deep and dark places that eating disorders take people to."

– **Marcella Raimondo, PhD**, Eating Disorder Therapist

"Dr. Fabello's work validates women's experiences of touch, intimacy, and their bodies, and does so in a way that researchers and academics can understand. She reveals a long-concealed narrative that is told about women who survive eating disorders and does so with their voices at the center. Every professional who works with women who experience problems with their eating should read this to learn how to better think about and talk to women about their bodies, their sex lives, and the relationships they want to have with others."

– **Justin A. Sitron, PhD**, Director of the Center for Human Sexuality Studies, Widener University

Appetite

The first comprehensive resource on anorexia and women's sexuality in the world, this book presents a model for understanding sexuality as complex with interconnected factors, and how anorexia interacts with the varied components of one's sexuality.

Challenging the limiting views of sexuality that research on women with anorexia and sex has yielded, Dr. Fabello centers real women's narratives to explore the various ways in which this population wrestles with sexual health, violence, intimacy, identity, and more. Included is unprecedented research on how women's level of desire for sensual touch interacts with body image, body perception, and a unique need for sexual autonomy.

Written in an honest voice, *Appetite* bridges the gap between academia and practicality, using grounded language that appeals to professionals and survivors alike.

Melissa A. Fabello, PhD, is a writer, educator, and researcher whose work focuses on the politics of bodies, relationships, and sexuality. She holds a doctorate in Human Sexuality Studies.

Appetite

Sex, Touch, and Desire in Women with Anorexia

Melissa A. Fabello

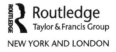

Routledge
Taylor & Francis Group

NEW YORK AND LONDON

First published 2021
by Routledge
52 Vanderbilt Avenue, New York, NY 10017

and by Routledge
2 Park Square, Milton Park, Abingdon, Oxon, OX14 4RN

Routledge is an imprint of the Taylor & Francis Group, an informa business

© 2021 Taylor & Francis

Library of Congress Cataloging-in-Publication Data
Names: Fabello, Melissa A., author.
Title: Appetite: sex, touch, and desire in women with anorexia /
Melissa A. Fabello.
Description: New York, NY: Routledge, 2021. |
Identifiers: LCCN 2020022405 (print) | LCCN 2020022406 (ebook) |
ISBN 9780367904098 (hardback) | ISBN 9780367904081 (paperback) |
ISBN 9781003024262 (ebook)
Subjects: LCSH: Anorexia nervosa—Patients—Sexual behavior. |
Women—Sexual behavior.
Classification: LCC RC552.A5 F33 2020 (print) |
LCC RC552.A5 (ebook) | DDC 616.85/262—dc23
LC record available at https://lccn.loc.gov/2020022405
LC ebook record available at https://lccn.loc.gov/2020022406

ISBN: 978-0-367-90409-8 (hbk)
ISBN: 978-0-367-90408-1 (pbk)
ISBN: 978-1-003-02426-2 (ebk)

Typeset in Calvert
by codeMantra

To those for whom this book offers puzzle pieces they never thought would fit.

Contents

Acknowledgments

Writing a dissertation – or a book based on your dissertation – is mostly a solitary endeavor. You have peers and advisors who celebrate and challenge you, but you're mostly stuck feeling like you're in a hell that no one understands. Here's a toast to those who made me feel less alone.

First and foremost, words cannot express my gratitude for those 20 who participated in my study, whose experiences splash color onto these pages. This project couldn't have been completed without your vulnerability and authenticity. More so, the hours of conversations we had affirmed a part of me buried so deep, I didn't recognize its cries for validation.

Thank you to my dissertation committee – a group that I put together specifically because I knew that they would both hold and push me. To my chair, Dr. Justin Sitron, who has made me a better researcher, educator, and person. To Dr. Don Dyson, for always finding a way to ask hard questions wrapped in generosity. To Dr. Marcella Raimondo, whose excitement for this project was always palpable and who gave me faith that this work matters.

To my cohorts at the Center for Human Sexuality Studies: I could never have made it through this process without venting over brunches, lunches, and cocktails with other people who understood what I was going through.

To my friends and cheerleaders in the field – the likes of Dr. Lindo Bacon, Jes Baker, Sonya Renee Taylor, Sam Dylan Finch, Sonalee Rashatwar, and more – who remind me every day how desperately necessary this work is. Especially to Gina Susanna, whose friendship is a gift from heaven. I wanted to write my first book without any help from anybody, but I guess that plan's moot: Gina, you make every day better. To *everyone*, really, who I have worked with over the years in the pursuits of social justice, body liberation, and especially eating disorder recovery advocacy: The communities that you have created and your commitment to changing the course of the world give me hope for tomorrow.

To my family – Mom, Dad, Rico, and Britt: You teach me new ways to understand the world around me every single day.

Especially to my partners, Imran Siddiquee and Tristan Guarini, whose daily validation of my brilliance and celebration of my accomplishments pushed me through every existential crisis a project like this can bring on. I wake up thankful for your love every single day.

And to Halley Amadeus, Astra Grace, and Vita Cornelia, who not only make me laugh, but also know to cuddle me when I'm crying.

To my team at Routledge, who has been nothing but supportive.

Lastly, to my beautiful and dedicated audience. Whether you're new to my work or have been following me for a decade, you give me a shining sense of purpose. No matter where I go and what I do, it will always be for you.

About the Author

Melissa A. Fabello, PhD, is a feminist writer, educator, and researcher whose work focuses on the politics of bodies, relationships, and sexuality. She received her PhD in Human Sexuality Studies from Widener University, where her phenomenological research explored how women with anorexia nervosa make meaning of their experiences with sensual touch. Melissa also holds an M.Ed. in Human Sexuality from Widener and a B.S. in English Education from Boston University. Previously, she worked as Managing Editor of Everyday Feminism, a social justice education platform. There, she accepted the Sex Ed in Media Award alongside founder, Sandra Kim, from the Center for Sex Education. She lives in Philadelphia with her partners and cats. Learn more at melissafabello.com. Follow her on Twitter and Instagram @fyeahmfabello.

Preface

I came into this work accidentally, believe it or not. When I started my doctoral program in Human Sexuality Studies, I didn't set out to write a dissertation on the experiences of touch in women with anorexia nervosa. The idea just came to me when, while preparing a literature review for another topic at the intersection of eating disorders and sexuality, I recognized that how much depth was missing from the conversation, specifically around sensuality: *Wait a minute. We know that women with anorexia tend to be sexually averse, but why isn't anyone asking about their experiences with sensual touch?* I was told once that you shouldn't start a research project – shouldn't even apply to a doctoral program – until you've encountered a question that hasn't been answered. This was mine.

Upon finishing my dissertation, and therefore my PhD, I made the conscious choice to make what I learned available to the masses. Instead of taking the usual route, working to have my work published by academic journals, I created an ebook that detailed my research. Important as it felt to have my work in the hands of academics, where it could be translated into practice and expanded upon in research, my social justice politics pushed me to first focus on the people: the sufferers, survivors, activists, and practitioners within the eating disorder space. I was proud, as a digital content creator, to produce something so unique to my interests and so necessary in the field. And the response was amazing: With over 1,000 downloads from all over the world and love notes thanking me for putting the experience of so many into words, I felt that I had accomplished exactly what I set out to do.

And now, that ebook has been revised and rereleased as the book that you hold now in your hands – finally making its way into academia proper, where I hope it will be given a whole new life. Academia is a complicated institution. It's marred by white supremacy, patriarchy, capitalism, and colonization. It's an arena in which rules and regulations can actually hinder, rather than foster, intellectual growth. The purpose of academia is to keep itself in power. As such, most academics sit in ivory tower echo chambers, sharing their work mostly, if not solely, with one another, competing to be the most brilliant in the room. However, to stay stuck on this aspect of academia is to ignore the radical shifts that feminist, queer, disability, and race theories, among others, have brought to this world. The idea that we can bend the bars of the academy – by committing ourselves to work within our own communities in ways that innately call into question the power-over dominance of traditional research – is one that too few people reach for. There are ways to push the boundaries of what is considered academically sound. My hope is that, by picking up this book that focuses on aspects of eating disorders and sexuality oft ignored, you are already that kind of changemaker.

My dissertation research, as well as this book, isn't astoundingly radical. There are many choices I could have made that would have made it more so – and perhaps, had I more time and money in this endeavor, I would have. But within the limitations with which I was working, I tried my best to infuse radical ideology. I chose to do a qualitative, phenomenological inquiry that prioritized the lived experiences of women, as told by them. I chose to engage in maximum diversity sampling, selecting participants based on the variety of perspectives they offered through social location and eating disorder experience. I chose to pay my participants for their narratives out of pocket, as I worked without grants, despite that being incredibly rare in qualitative research. And I wrote a digital book before I even entertained the thought of being published more widely, in order to bring my findings to people on the ground. I wanted this work to be representative of my perspective on the world and on academia: I wanted to look at a problem clinically minute, yet hugely influential on women's lives; I wanted to show how powerful it can be for those affected to see someone like them focus on an issue brushed off by everyone else. I wanted to demonstrate how using a social justice lens can only benefit research.

Within these pages, then, you will find a labor of love. I could only commit to this years-long project because I was passionate about it. And I could only produce this book because people like you were, too.

Introduction

Chapter 1

Simply put, this book is a re-exploration of the intersection of eating disorders and sexuality specifically from a sexological purview – that is, a perspective that centers the biological, psychological, and sociocultural phenomena within sexuality. Most of the research that looks at sexuality in eating disorder populations is done by clinical psychologists, and bless them for that. But because inquiries into sexuality are being published by psychologists and not sexologists, there's some nuance missing from the conversation that could be helpful in connecting dots. Part of what I tried to do with my dissertation research, and therefore in this book, is to shine a sex researcher's light onto the work that's being done in this field.

I received my PhD in Human Sexuality Studies from Widener University in 2018, after spending four years working on a phenomenological approach to understanding the experiences women with anorexia nervosa have with skin hunger (the extent to which we crave sensual interaction). I studied touch and sensuality specifically, as I wondered how those experiences held up against the common knowledge that this population is more sexually averse. In order to explore the specific phenomenon of skin hunger, however, I first had to understand, in depth, how this population interacts with sexuality on various planes. Chapter 2 of my dissertation, the literature review (also known as the bane of my existence), contains almost 100 pages. That is the foundation of this book.

This book, then, at its core, is a literature review. In my dissertation, I used the Circles of Sexuality (more on that later) as a model for breaking down the vast complexity of sexuality, and in my literature review, I visited each of the components of that model. I took most of what I wrote there and reworked it into this book, toning down the academic jargon, adding editorialized context, and working in the insights I gained from the interviews I conducted in my own study. As such, it is research-heavy, but hopefully entertaining as it is educational. The pro is that the book serves as a comprehensive survey of what we know, academically, about women with anorexia nervosa and sexuality. The con is that traditional research is only one way to explore a topic – and in many ways, research can be harmful in how it is conducted and in who it leaves out.

In my work – and thus, in this book – I focused specifically on women with anorexia nervosa. This was a difficult choice to make. Most research on eating disorders is done with this population in mind, and I didn't want to add to this dominance. However, I had to limit my work *somehow*, and I decided to focus on this population for two reasons: (1) Because in looking at an intersection so shallowly covered, the most research existed on this population for me to draw from, and (2) because I, myself, identify as a woman with (or in recovery from) anorexia nervosa. It made sense to me to engage in intracommunity work, from a feminist research perspective, and this also gave me the opportunity to work with the most information at hand. In the future, I hope to have the opportunity to expand this work to incorporate more genders and eating disorder experiences.

What, though, does "woman with anorexia nervosa" really mean? The research and I largely disagree. *For me*, it means any person who identifies as a woman exhibiting symptoms in line with those of all anorexia nervosa diagnoses. Restrictive and binge/purge subtypes, of course, are included in that definition – but in my own work, I also make a point to include the Other Specified Feeding and Eating Disorders (OSFED) diagnosis of atypical anorexia, specifically because it allows people with anorexia symptoms who are *not* underweight access to participation, where they are almost always left out. In my work, I also allow folks to self-identify, rather than to be required to hold an official medical diagnosis, an unfortunately radical choice within the social sciences. Diagnoses are often only available to people with more access to healthcare, and requiring them limits the pool considerably. Further, I want to fight back against the misconception that eating disorders are the realm of white, thin, able, cisgender women; it was important to me that I interview women with various identities and experiences. While most of the participants in my own dissertation study were cisgender women, I also interviewed two transgender, three non-binary, and two intersex women. I purposely included women who were diverse in age, race, sexual identity, ability, income, and size, as well as in eating disorder experience. My participants were 70% of color, 85% queer, 60% disabled, 60% poor and working class, 20% fat or plus-size, and 70% in recovery. I want you to remember this for an important reason: Throughout the book, I sprinkle in my own participants' narrative experiences. When you see their words, remember that they largely do *not* represent the most privileged groups. This is partially to mitigate the limited purview of the other research that I quote.

Unfortunately, the aforementioned choices are uncommon in eating disorder research. Often, researchers don't expound upon what "woman with anorexia nervosa" means to them. While data is sometimes collected on diagnosis, age, or race, most identities are left out of the conversation entirely, unless the research is identity-focused. This leaves us to assume the worst, from a social justice standpoint: that most of the research being done on eating disorders and sexuality is conducted using participants from the most privileged backgrounds. This is an astounding limitation. When I quote research throughout this book on "women with anorexia nervosa," take liberty to assume that samples aren't diverse – and as such, results are not necessarily generalizable. I do not, by any means, want you to assume my stamp of approval on the sampling methods of the research herein; I'm simply offering you what is available, with all of the limitations that this entails. It is my sincere intention, over the course of my academic career, to assist in adding to this body of desperately needed knowledge.

Another issue that we come across in eating disorder research is time. According to the National Institute of Health (2015), eating disorder research received approximately $30 million in grants, contracts, and other funding mechanisms for research in 2014. But with prevalence estimated at 30 million people in the United States suffering from clinically significant eating disorders (Wade, Keski-Rahkonen, & Hudson, 2011), this funding amounts to one dollar per individual affected. Eating disorder research isn't receiving a whole lot of funding these days. And funding that *is* available tends to favor research working to uncover biological determinants for eating disorders. Important as those studies are, it also means that research exploring eating disorders and sexuality isn't particularly hot right now – and hasn't been for quite some time. As such, you'll notice that many of the studies quoted throughout this book come from the 1990s – a time when eating disorder panic was high and more funding was offered to explore what now might feel like minutia. Citing older studies is generally considered academically inappropriate; however, as it's considered sound to quote older research in situations in which further research hasn't been established, I've taken liberty to use that foundational research here.

Academic research is not only flawed, which we can all admit to readily. It is also an active oppressive force – and always has been. Research has always been used to support the status quo, and the history of eating disorder research is no different. From suffering women being dismissed as "hysterical" to the active exclusion of marginalized groups to the lack of sociopolitical underpinnings in the research, our understanding of these complex disorders has always chiefly been from the perspective of white men with social, economic, and political power, treating white, thin, upper-middle-class, cisgender women. What follows is not (and can't ever be) the be all, end all of the conversation; it is only one entry point. Especially because most of the research quoted herein is quantitative – that is, lacking the goal of listening to, interpreting, and reporting on stories – it can only take us so far in understanding. Reading research is useful for gaining a cursory view of trends, which is what I hope to offer here. But it is never a substitute for listening to the lived experiences of those with eating disorders – and taking their subjective narratives as truths in and of themselves.

It is my hope that this book offers you something to chew on – and that the digestion of this information, over time, will lead you to continue to explore this intersection in rich and rewarding ways. I hope that it offers you some solace, some validation, and some affirmation first and foremost – but also some information along the way.

Let's get started.

REFERENCES

National Institute of Health. (2015). *Estimates of funding for various research, condition, and disease categories (RCDC)*. Retrieved from http://report.nih.gov/categorical_spending.aspx

Wade, T.D., Keski-Rahkonen, A., & Hudson, J. (2011). Epidemiology of eating disorders. In M. Tsuang & M. Tohen (Eds.), *Textbook in psychiatric epidemiology* (3rd ed., pp. 343–360). New York, NY: Wiley.

Defining Women with Anorexia

Chapter 2

We run into a serious problem when we endeavor to research the experiences of women with anorexia nervosa: The bulk of the research is done on a homogenous population of white, middle-to-upper class women, most of whom are also straight, cisgender, thin, and, mental health notwithstanding, abled. And to put it bluntly: That simply does not encapsulate the generalizable experiences of women. If we only look at the lived experience of *some* women, our research only reflects that group.

"Due to our historically biased view that eating disorders only affect" this group (National Eating Disorders Association, 2015a, para. 1), there is a lack of accurate, diverse information on the prevalence and effects of eating disorders. And this lack of inclusion can have devastating effects for marginalized populations, who suffer from eating disorders, including anorexia nervosa, at similar rates to the population dominant in research. Without information on marginalized groups – without including an anti-oppression analysis in research – we are stunningly unable to understand, never mind assist, people who belong to those groups, especially those for whom oppressions overlap.

Y'all. That's not good. That is, plain and simple, injustice.

Because the literature quoted within this book mostly reflects research conducted with a population of more privileged women (those who are white, middle-to-upper class, with access to healthcare, and so on), we first need to contextualize that: This research does not reflect the experiences of all women. In fact, various social locations – like wealth, race, dis/ability, age, and size – deeply impact how eating disorders are experienced.

With the understanding that intersectionality makes these relationships incredibly complex (Crenshaw, 1989), let's look at how anorexia nervosa shows up for groups historically excluded in eating disorder research.

WEALTH AND ACCESS

When we talk about wealth and access, we don't just mean money – although that's a huge, underlying factor. Wealth also indicates access to opportunities and resources. Healthcare, here in the United States, is a great example. Because healthcare is tied to employment, and because salaried, as compared to hourly waged, jobs come with higher pay, those with more access to wealth *also* incur more access to healthcare. This makes wealth a significant social determinant of health.

According to the World Health Organization (2016, para. 1), social determinants of health are "the conditions in which people are born, grow, live, work, and age." These forces and systems include economics, development, social norms and policies, and political systems, and these "circumstances are shaped by the distribution of money, power, and resources." Social determinants of health are the sociocultural factors that play a role in our quality of life, where those who are the most disenfranchised are the ones most disadvantaged. And, also according to the World Health Organization (2016), these oppressive injustices are what are "mostly responsible for health inequities."

According to the Centers for Disease Control and Prevention (2016), there are five determinants of population health: Genes/biology, health behaviors, social environment, physical environment, and access to health services. We often consider our genes (or overall biology) and health-supportive behaviors to be significant determiners of health outcomes, but in actuality, they only account for approximately 25% of population health. The three remaining categories of population health – social environment, physical environment, and access to health services and medical care – much more highly determine our individual and group health. That is to say, the likelihood is that the more access you have, through social location, the healthier you'll be.

Wealth and access, frequently referred to in the literature as *socioeconomic status (SES)*, is a question of an individual's financial situation, which includes how that relates to their ability to obtain health-related resources. And there has long been an assumption that eating disorders are associated with middle-to-upper class women (Maresh & Willard, 1996). But this may not actually be true: In a review of the literature on SES and eating disorders, Gard and Freeman (1995) explored the research that was available to them at the time, spanning from the early 1970s through the early 1990s. And they concluded that the stereotype that those more likely to develop eating disorders are of higher SES could not be confirmed. The relationship between anorexia nervosa and higher SES was assumed, but not empirically proven, they said. And, in fact, there was increasing evidence to suggest the *opposite* relationship in regard to bulimia nervosa: that those with less access were more likely to develop that eating disorder.

Similarly, in 1997, Rogers, Resnick, Mitchell, and Blum explored the potential relationship between SES and self-reported eating disorder behavior in a group of adolescent women and found *none*. They did find a relationship between unhealthy dieting behaviors and higher SES, similar to other studies (Story, French, Resnick, & Blum, 1995), as well as a relationship between weight and SES – that higher SES can predict thinness, also echoing prior research (Iancu, Spivak, Ratzoni, Apter, & Weizman, 1994; Osvald & Sodowsky, 1993). But this may be related to a history of those with more wealth being more likely to fit the social standard of health and beauty at the time, due to having more leisure time and access to resources to obtain and attain the bodies associated with wealth (Gerber, 2011).

This prevailing assumption that eating disorders are more likely to occur in people with more wealth and access is dangerous, though, because it affects diagnosis and treatment. Maresh and Willard (1996, p. 96) noted, for instance, that anorexia nervosa may be "overlooked in a population in which weight loss is frequently assumed to result from malnutrition" – like in those who are poor and working class – and may, therefore, be undiagnosed. Also, because other psychiatric diagnoses are more commonly associated with poverty, such as substance abuse and schizophrenia, these diagnoses may be misapplied to people with less wealth and access instead (Maresh & Willard, 1996).

Maresh and Willard (1996, p. 96) wrote, "The lack of social and professional resources available to this type of patient presents additional impediments to comprehensive, effective treatment," especially in regard to the current political attitudes toward healthcare. The "fiscally driven viewpoint" on long-term psychotherapy, for instance, is that it is "both unnecessary and ineffective" (Maresh & Willard, 1996, p. 99), which further solidifies it as an option only for those with enough wealth and access to circumvent financial and social barriers to healthcare.

Women who are middle-to-upper class are not only more likely to recognize eating disorder behavior in themselves, and have that behavior acknowledged by others as well, but are also more likely to receive diagnoses and treatment for those eating disorders. And while *surely*, they deserve that care, doesn't everyone?

Mythical theories on SES "continue to guide and inform research" and are "frequently translated into…treatment" (Gard & Freeman, 1995, p. 11). This creates a system that will always exclude society's most vulnerable from accessing the support that they need, especially when their access is complicated by other social intersections of marginalization.

RACE

Similar to wealth and how eating disorders are assumed to be the domain of middle-to-upper class women, there is also a pervasive myth that eating disorders only affect white women (Dolan, 1989; National Eating Disorders Association, 2015a). That Stephanie Covington Armstrong titled her 2009 memoir about bulimia *Not All Black Girls Know How to Eat* says a lot about how deeply held our beliefs are around race and eating disorders.

But this myth – that women of color are immune to eating disorders – is false. The truth is that eating disorder prevalence in the United States is similar across racial and ethnic backgrounds, only with the exception of anorexia nervosa, which is more commonly diagnosed (though not necessarily experienced) in white people (Hudson, Hiripi, Pope, & Kessler, 2007; Wade, Keski-Rahkonen, & Hudson, 2011). Yet, as Dolan (1989) points out, within eating disorder research, "it is noticeable that the issues of culture, race, and ethnicity are lost in the small print of results sections or given only passing mention in discussions," even though race and ethnicity are "surely among the most powerful sociocultural variables existing" (p. 67).

Dieting, which can often trigger or lead to eating disorders (Shisslak, Crago, & Estes, 1995), is associated with weight dissatisfaction, the negative perception of being fat, and negative body image similarly across all racial and ethnic groups (Blum et al., 1988; Neumark-Sztainer, Story, Resnick, & Blum, 1998). Asian, Black, and Latinx adolescents report attempts to lose weight at similar rates to white youth, while Indigenous adolescents attempt weight loss at the highest rate: 48% report engaging in this behavior (Kilpatrick, Ohannessian, & Bartholomew, 1999). In fact, among the thinnest quarter of sixth- and seventh-grade girls, Latina and Asian girls report more body dissatisfaction than any other racial or ethnic group, including white girls (Robinson et al., 1996).

This information can be surprising to some, who wrongfully believe that women of color are protected from eating disorder development by virtue of their cultural identity and the body types and eating habits assumed to be embraced in those communities (National Eating Disorders Association, 2015a). The publication of research that suggests that women of color experience eating disorders at the same rates of their white peers, then, might lead some to wonder if eating disorders are on the rise in this population. But the National Eating Disorders Association (2015a) suggests that there is simply a rise in people of color *reporting* eating disorders. Traditionally, there have been several reasons for lower rates of reporting among people of color: According to the National Eating Disorders Association (2015a, para. 4), these reasons include "underreporting of problems by the individual, under- and misdiagnosing on the part of the treatment provider, and cultural bias…[against] criteria for eating disorders."

Also, eating disorder symptoms present differently in various communities of color (Alegria et al., 2007; Tareen, Hodes, & Rangel, 2005). The problem is that how we conceptualize eating disorders is based on a white prototype. According to Alegria et al. (2007), who explored eating disorder prevalence among Latinx people in the United States, "[s]tandard eating disorder criteria may not be appropriate for understanding psychological morbidity for eating disorders" in marginalized racial and ethnic groups (p. S15). As Tareen et al. (2005), who investigated anorexia nervosa in South Asian adolescent women in Britain, explained, "Differing symptom profiles for anorexia nervosa need to be taken into account when assessing patients from different cultures" – that is, those outside of the dominant group (p. 161).

In *A Hunger So Wide and So Deep: A Multiracial View of Women's Eating Problems*, Thompson (1994) relays the information she gathered from interviewing 18 women of various marginalized identities, including race and ethnicity. She found that eating disorders often developed as a response to environmental stress that the women were subjected to, including various forms of abuse, racism, and poverty. Thompson suggests that these multiple traumas, to which many women of color are exposed, may affect the rate of eating disorder development in this group.

In the case of eating disorders, one specific manifestation of white supremacist oppression worth exploring is beauty ideals. Feminists have long argued that cultural beauty standards, as affected by patriarchy, are narrowly defined (Wolf, 2002). However, at their intersection with race, beauty standards can have a compounded effect on women of color. Hall (1995) noted that those who are furthest from the dominant beauty ideal, "specifically women of color, may suffer the psychological effects of low self-esteem, poor body image, and eating disorders" (p. 8). Why? Because cultural beauty standards aren't only focused on thinness, but also on whiteness (among other factors). Because women of color are multiply marginalized, they're also multiply striving toward an unrealistic ideal. As women of color, particularly those who are immigrants, acculturate or assimilate to dominant cultural ideals, they can become more vulnerable to eating disorders as a coping mechanism (National Eating Disorders Association, 2015a).

According to Kempa and Thomas (2000), this relationship is dependent on the stage of ethnic identity of the individual. They explain that if a person is in the conformity stage (Phinney, 1989), wherein they tend to be self-deprecating toward the self and appreciative of the dominant group, they may be more likely to internalize the dominant culture's beauty ideals. This is a state that could potentially lead to eating disorders. But if they're in the dissonance stage (Phinney, 1989), wherein they're in conflict as to whether to appreciate the self or the dominant group, they may actually be more sensitive to oppression, and therefore potentially more likely to develop eating disorders as a coping mechanism (Kempa & Thomas, 2000). It's possible that as people move toward more comfort with the self and more questioning of the dominant culture (Phinney, 1989), they may be more likely to *reject* those ideals and be *less* likely to develop eating disorders.

The more strongly a person identifies with their culture of origin, the less likely they may be to internalize American beauty ideals: Jane, Hunter, and Lozzi (1999) found that Cuban-American women had less negative attitudes toward eating the more closely they associated with Cuban culture. Similarly, Lake, Staiger, and Glowinski (2000) found that Australians born in Hong Kong were less likely to express body dissatisfaction than those of Hong Kong descent born in Australia. Chamorro and Flores-Ortiz (2000) found that second-generation Mexican-American women, those who were born to immigrant parents, had high eating disorder patterns; similarly, Osvald and Sodowsky (1993) found that the more accepting of white American culture that Black and Indigenous women were, the more symptoms of anorexia and bulimia nervosas they showed.

Eating disorders are not less prevalent in communities of color; if anything, they crop up largely as a response to oppression. They simply go unnoticed because how we've been trained to recognize eating disorders is specific to white women.

DIS/ABILITY

Despite anorexia nervosa, as a mental illness, arguably being a disability unto itself, research exploring co-occurrences of disability and eating disorders is extremely limited, aside from how eating disorders interact with other mental health issues.

Partially, this is because of a long-standing assumption that the presence of a physical disability is somehow a protective factor against negative body image and weight control behaviors. If you're sensing a theme here, it's because it's painfully obvious: We assume that experiences of marginalization somehow prevent eating disorders, rather than understanding that what we're looking for might be different. Similar to race and class, disability isn't a protective factor either.

In fact, in 2000, Gross, Ireys, and Kinsman found that young women with specific physical disabilities (in this case, spina bifida and arthritis) reported anorexia and bulimia symptomology at *higher* rates than the general population. And maybe this should come as no surprise because in eating disorder populations, women are more likely to have experienced another physical illness *prior* to the onset of their eating disorder. And this might suggest that physical illness could actually be a risk factor for the development of anorexia nervosa in particular (Patton, Wood, & Johnson-Sabine, 1986; Watkins, Sutton, & Lask, 2001). For example, adolescents with chronic illnesses that include a dietary component – like type

1 diabetes, cystic fibrosis, celiac disease, inflammatory bowel diseases, and irritable bowel syndrome – "may be at risk of adopting disordered eating practices that can develop into a full-blown eating disorder over the course of their treatment" (Quick, Byrd-Bredbenner, & Neumark-Sztainer, 2013, p. 282).

One possible explanation for this is that the eating disorder behavior is connected to the experience of physical disability in and of itself. Smith, Latchford, Hall, and Dickson (2008) suggest that restrictive eating in their sample of 76 women with scoliosis may have been motivated by a desire to minimize the ways in which their disorder impacts their appearance. That is, potentially, women with both physical disabilities and eating disorders are less motivated specifically by weight control and more motivated by the effects of their disability. In fact, disabled women are more likely to report eating disorder symptoms if they have multiple co-existing conditions or experience feelings of uncertainty in regard to their illness(es) (Gross, Ireys, & Kinsman, 2000). This might suggest that women with physical disabilities may develop eating disorders as a way to cope with their disorders.

Indeed, among other factors – such as social support, media literacy, and a broad conception of beauty – a woman's acceptance of her disability contributes to positive body image (Bailey, Gammage, van Ingen, & Ditor, 2015). And this includes some disability-specific bodily appreciations, such as functional gains, independence, managing secondary complications, and minimizing pain. This is important, considering that women with physical disabilities have prevalence rates of body dissatisfaction similar to or higher than non-disabled women (Pinquart, 2012; Spitzer, Henderson, & Zivian, 1999), a dissatisfaction not limited to the body parts that are affected by their disability (Gross et al., 2000).

When we turn to psychological disorders, we find that general personality traits, as well as so-called personality pathology, are often at the center of research around eating disorders, and especially anorexia nervosa: It's been suggested that certain dispositions are more likely to be susceptible to eating disorder development. For example, high levels of obsessionality, restraint, and perfectionism have been associated with people with anorexia nervosa (Wonderlich, Lilenfeld, Riso, Engel, & Mitchell, 2005). The same population has also been determined to experience high levels of stimulus-seeking behavior, self-harm, oppositionality, and compulsivity (Lavender et al., 2013).

Furthermore, 97% of women with eating disorders experience one or more comorbid diagnosis (Blinder, Cumella, & Sanathara, 2006): In one study, 94% of participants experienced mood disorders (most significantly, depression), 56% experienced anxiety disorders, and 22% experienced substance use disorders, which was twice as likely in women with bulimia nervosa (Blinder et al., 2006). Women with the restrictive subtype of anorexia nervosa were twice as likely to experience obsessive-compulsive disorder and three times as likely to experience schizophrenia and other psychoses; women with the binge/purge subtype of anorexia nervosa were twice as likely to experience obsessive-compulsive disorder, twice as likely to experience post-traumatic stress disorder, and twice as likely to experience schizophrenia and other psychoses.

Depression is especially relevant to sexuality research in the realm of eating disorders: Depression, which is commonly comorbid with anorexia nervosa, is frequently found to have a strong effect on sexual functioning and expression (Godart et al., 2006, 2007). Approximately 70% of people with eating disorders will develop depressive symptomology, and only one-third of them will experience depression prior to the manifestation of the eating disorder (Fernández-Aranda et al., 2007). Because of the pathophysiology of depression, as well as the side effects of various medications used to treat it, depression has been shown to have a strong adverse effect on sexual functioning (Reynaert, Zdanowicz, Janne, & Jacques, 2010). For this reason, it's unknown whether women with both anorexia nervosa and depression experience issues with sexuality because of the former, the latter, or both.

When we look at cognitive functioning, we find that learning disabilities in people with eating disorders have been explored less frequently. But research suggests that some people with learning disabilities show both the emotional and cognitive characteristics of typical eating disorders (Jones & Samuel, 2010). In fact, one 2004 study by Hove found that 27% of people with learning disabilities had eating disorders, with binge eating disorder being the most common manifestation. In this study, anorexia nervosa was associated with more severe learning disabilities. However, in 2007, Hove published results looking at the same sample, but exploring eating behaviors more generally, rather than eating disorder diagnostic criteria, and found that 64% of this sample showed dysfunctional eating behavior.

According to Felstrom, Mulryan, Reidy, and Hillery (2005), disordered eating in people with learning disabilities can include a wider range of behaviors than what's assessed for in general populations. While restricting, bingeing, and purging are more commonly understood as potential eating disorder symptomology, people with learning disabilities may be more likely to engage in pica (the ingestion of non-food items) and rumination (regurgitation and rechewing of food) (Jones & Samuel, 2010). Pica has been named the most common disordered eating behavior in people with learning disabilities (Danford & Huber, 1981), and rumination is thought to occur in 5–10% of adults who have been institutionalized and is more common in people with severe learning disabilities (Gravestock, 2000). These behaviors are sometimes misclassified as disorders of infancy in this population; instead, "eating problems, if not disorders, are significant" in people with learning disabilities (Jones & Samuel, 2010, p. 363).

A question that deserves more exploration in this field is whether or not anorexia nervosa, in and of itself, should be considered a disability. According to Tierney (2001), the oppression that people with anorexia nervosa experience mirrors that of ableist oppression, yet it isn't generally considered a disability because of the "narrow social understanding" of the term *disability* (p. 743). The general public often reserves this term to describe people with physical disabilities, especially those that are visible. The social model of disability (Oliver, 1983), which locates disability in society, rather than in the individual, could be a useful tool for people with anorexia nervosa looking to better understand their experiences. According to the social model of disability, systemic barriers and oppressive attitudes are what "disable" people. Variations in physicality, senses, intellect, and psychology aren't inherently disabling; a society that doesn't consider those differences in the building of institutions and infrastructure is what creates limitations. Identifying systemic barriers to care and individual and social stereotypes, prejudice, and discrimination are the chief issues that people with anorexia nervosa face, rather than their supposed own inability to function "normally" in society, could be helpful, both individually and socially.

   According to Tierney (2001), claiming the identity of disability could be helpful for people with anorexia nervosa in the following ways: People with anorexia nervosa could claim benefits if unable to work; anorexia nervosa might be treated more seriously; it would "emphasize the fact that… it is in a state of flux" (p. 753), while also highlighting its longevity; and it could help elucidate the oppression that people with anorexia nervosa face. Yet, according to Tierney's 2001 qualitative study on how women with anorexia nervosa feel about being labeled disabled, most participants were uncomfortable with the identity. In fact, only one participant involved in the interviews identified as disabled already. The participants explained that they felt that the term *disability* was linked to the experience of physical limitations and was associated with permanence. They also explained that they felt that identifying as disabled would limit "one's life opportunities," partly because they believed that by identifying as disabled, they would be assuming the role of the victim, a common experience in disabled people (Peters, 1996, p. 754). Tierney (2001) pointed out that disabled people and people with anorexia nervosa "face social oppression because of their 'difference' from a culture that demands conformity, which is fixated with aesthetic and behavioral 'norms'" – and that because of this similarity, adopting the social model of disability as a lens through which to explore eating disorders could be useful (p. 755).

AGE

Age is often a conversation left out of social justice analysis entirely. Within eating disorder research – and even just conceptualization – the same problem exists: We practically forget that older people exist – and are vulnerable. The stereotypical woman living with an eating disorder is a young one; however, in reality, more older women than ever are seeking support for disordered thoughts and behaviors around food (National Eating Disorders Association, 2015b). In fact, in 2003, one-third of inpatient psychiatric admissions for eating disorders were women over 30 (Maine & Kelly, 2005). Despite the fact that the medically ideal body weight for maximum life expectancy increases with advancing age (Soenen & Chapman, 2013), the experience of body dissatisfaction for people in midlife more than doubled between 1972 and 1997 – to more than half of the population (Garner, 1997).

Women aged 61 through 92 name weight as their greatest bodily concern (Clarke, 2002), some harboring these issues from their youth, and some being triggered by aging. Unsurprisingly, this, in part, leads to over 20% of women 70 and older dieting (Berg, 2001). Embarrassed by their affliction's association with youth, older women experience more difficulty admitting their need for help. According to the National Eating Disorders Association (2015b), "Contemporary women experience unprecedented stress due to: their rapidly changing role in a globalized consumer culture; the strict cultural standards regarding women, weight, and appearance; unattainable media images"; and a fear of fat. Because of these stressors, some older women find comfort in the "body myth" (Maine & Kelly, 2005): the idea that achieving the ideal body will improve their worth. Especially in a culture that values youth and where women are aged out of society at a faster rate, older adult women may turn to destructive habits to help them cope. As older women experience potentially triggering life events – such as menopause, signs of aging, death, empty nest, and becoming grandparents (National Eating Disorders Association, 2015b) – they become more vulnerable to developing symptoms of anorexia nervosa, an illness with medical complications that can be especially dangerous for older populations.

The exploration of anorexia (not anorexia nervosa, the psychological disorder, but the symptomatic lack of appetite associated with various medical and psychological issues) in older populations, however, isn't new. As people grow older, a complex interplay of biological, psychological, and sociocultural factors may influence their developing a lack of appetite known as *anorexia of aging* (Martone et al., 2013). Partly, this is due to the physiological processes that affect the experiences of satiation and satiety – such as gastric emptying and levels of gut hormones – which change as bodies age, leading to a lack of hunger cues (Benelam, 2009). And other physiological influences, such as poor dentition, ill-fitting dentures, and age-associated changes in taste and smell, can play a role, too (Donini, Savina, & Cannella, 2003). Moreover, poverty, loneliness, depression, and social isolation can also contribute to decreased food intake in this population (Donini et al., 2003). These factors can be dangerous, and "scientific evidence indicates that a significant number of frail elderly people fail to get the proper amount of food necessary to meet essential energy and nutrient needs" (Landi et al., 2010, p. 268). This can lead to various physical and mental impairments, including being underweight, malnourished, and at an increased risk of developing various diseases (Morley, 1997).

This weight loss, and its associated complications, is one of the most prevalent problems in older populations (Landi et al., 2000; Morley, 2007), as it's an individual predictor of morbidity and mortality for older adults (Cartwright, Hickman, Perrin, & Tilden, 2006; Kuh, 2007). Anorexia of aging may be a normal development in the average aging process; however, poor nutritional status, especially in terms of protein-energy malnutrition, can be very dangerous (Donini et al., 2003). As such, healthcare providers should screen older adults for this lack of appetite and should prioritize the integration of education in exercise and nutrition for this population (Visvanathan, 2015).

Arguably, anorexia of aging isn't directly related to eating disorder development in adults, but understanding of the former can lead to clearer diagnosis in and treatment of the latter.

SIZE

Body dissatisfaction and the drive for thinness are both well-known risk factors for eating disorder development (National Eating Disorders Association, 2015c). However, despite the fact that fat people (a phrase I use purposefully to destigmatize the word *fat*, as per the lead of radical fat activists) are perhaps more likely to be socialized into these traits, eating disorders among this population often go unrecognized (Bacon, 2010).

Partly, healthism plays a role in this. Healthism (Crawford, 1980), an oppressive system under which we value people presumed to be healthy more than those who aren't, creates a culture wherein the supposed aesthetics of health, like thinness, are valued. As such, people go to great lengths to achieve a body that they believe will increase their worth. Over the course of the past 70 years, according to Macpherson-Sánchez (2015, p. e71), "self-induced famine (dieting to achieve and maintain a lower weight)" has become a social norm in the United States. This has contributed to the widespread fear of gaining weight or becoming fat, which is seen in weight stigma through cognition, affect, and behavior from others (Ottati, Bodenhausen, & Newman, 2004) and self-stigma in fat people themselves (Corrigan & Kleinlein, 2004; Puhl, Moss-Racusin, & Schwartz, 2007). Even current, socially accepted health policies in regard to the so-called "obesity epidemic" support weight stigma (Vartanian & Smyth, 2013). It's perhaps no wonder, then, that fat people "may face unintended consequences of [these] well-intentioned interventions" (Miller, 2014, para. 10). This so-called "War on Obesity" might play into the development of eating disorders more generally speaking, but especially in those at whom these messages are directed (Miller, 2014).

Because of the cultural imperative, disguised as medical necessity, to lose weight, when fat people experience dramatic weight loss, even if through disordered eating behaviors, they're overlooked at best, and applauded at worst (Miller,

2014). The maintaining of low weight may be considered problematic and symptomatic in eating disorder literature, but in what is referred to as "obesity" research, low weight maintenance is considered virtuous (Macpherson-Sánchez, 2015). However, the dieting process in and of itself, which is frequently prescribed to fat people, may trigger an obsession with energy restriction and lead to an eating disorder (Miller, 2014). This creates a positive feedback cycle: When weight loss in fat people is celebrated in the name of health, these compliments reinforce the behaviors in which they're engaging to achieve that weight loss (Miller, 2014).

However, one's body mass index (BMI) is not an accurate marker of health, and the scale itself is flawed (Bacon, 2010). For example, as Miller (2014) quoted Sim as explaining, since BMI can't show how severe an eating disorder is, a person with an eating disorder can have a BMI in the 50th percentile, but be "sicker than [those] at the 10th percentile" (para. 16). The cultural preoccupation in the United States with treating the body as a project in need of constant improvement (Brumberg, 1998), though, oftentimes ignores the measures taken to achieve the cultural beauty ideal. This leads to eating disorder diagnosis being delayed an average of *nine months* in people with a history of being fat, compared with those who have never been fat (Sim, Lebow, & Billings, 2013). This, compounded with the fact that fat people "worry that they will be humiliated and rejected because of their weight" if they seek help for eating disorders (National Eating Disorders Association, 2015c, para. 2), creates a uniquely dangerous situation for this population.

It's been shown, in fact, that fat adolescents are just as likely to develop eating disorders as their non-fat counterparts (Sim et al., 2013). Some research even suggests that fat people often have eating disorders (Müller et al., 2012) and that being fat, in and of itself, is a risk factor for bulimia nervosa and binge eating disorder (de Zwaan, 2001). According to Villarejo et al. (2014), symptoms of bingeing and purging in fat people are "clinically relevant" (p. 25), as there are "significantly higher levels of eating symptomathology and general psychopathology" in fat populations who experience binge eating (p. 26).

However, while the relationship between being fat and experiencing bulimia nervosa or binge eating disorder has been established, fewer studies have explored the experience of anorexia nervosa in this population, even though being fat may be an antecedent to the disorder (Neumark-Sztainer, Story, Hannan, Perry, & Irving, 2002; Sim et al., 2013). In 2015, Lebow, Sim, and Kransdorf completed a retrospective cohort study of new clients seen in an eating disorder clinic. They looked specifically at 179 young people, aged 9 through 22, who had been diagnosed with anorexia nervosa or eating disorder not otherwise specified (EDNOS) characterized by weight loss and/or dietary restriction. What they found was that over one-third (36.7%) of these adolescents seeking treatment were at or above the 85th percentile for BMI. They also found that those with a history of being in this BMI category experienced a longer duration of their illness before presentation. The researchers concluded that "extreme weight loss in adolescents is not healthy, regardless of whether the end weight is theoretically within a healthy range" (p. 19).

And that's a line of thinking we would all do well to get behind.

Intersectional perspective in the exploration of eating disorders isn't just an important addition to the work; it's imperative to understanding. As we'll see unfold in this book, sexuality is made up of a complex web of identities and experiences. Social location doesn't escape that complexity. If anything, it should be centered.

REFERENCES

Alegria, M., Woo, M., Cao, Z., Torres, M., Meng, X., & Striegel-Moore, R. (2007). Prevalence and correlates of eating disorders in Latinos in the United States. *International Journal of Eating Disorders, 40*(Suppl), S15–S21. doi:10.1002/eat

Armstrong, S. C. (2009). *Not all black girls know how to eat: A story of bulimia.* Chicago, IL: Lawrence Hill Books.

Bacon, L. (2010). *Health at every size: The surprising truth about your weight* (2nd ed.). Dallas, TX: BenBella Books.

Bailey, K. A., Gammage, K. L., van Ingen, C., & Ditor, D. S. (2015). "It's all about acceptance": A qualitative study exploring a model of positive body image for people with spinal cord injury. *Body Image, 15*, 24–32. doi:10.1016/j.bodyim.2015.04.010

Defining Women with Anorexia

Benelam, B. (2009). Satiety and the anorexia of aging. *British Journal of Community Nursing, 14*(8), 332–335. Retrieved from http://www.ncbi.nlm.nih.gov/pubmed/19684553

Berg, F. M. (2001). *Women afraid to eat: Breaking free in today's weight-obsessed world.* Hettinger, ND: Healthy Weight Network.

Blinder, B. J., Cumella, E. J., & Sanathara, V. A. (2006). Psychiatric comorbidities of female inpatients with eating disorders. *Psychosomatic Medicine, 68*(3), 454–462. doi:10.1097/01.psy.0000221254.77675.f5

Blum, R. W., Geer, L., Hutton, L., McKay, C., Resnick, M. D., Rosenwinkel, K., & Song, Y. (1988). The Minnesota adolescent health survey: Implications for physicians. *Minnesota Medicine, 71*(3), 143–145, 149. Retrieved from http://www.ncbi.nlm.nih.gov/pubmed/3412266

Brumberg, J. J. (1998). *The body project: An intimate history of American girls.* New York, NY: Vintage Publishing.

Cartwright, J. C., Hickman, S., Perrin, N., & Tilden, V. (2006). Symptom experiences of residents dying in assisted living. *Journal of the American Medical Directors Association, 7*(4), 219–223. doi:10.1016/j.jamda.2005.09.011

Centers for Disease Control and Prevention. (2016). *Social determinants of health: Frequently asked questions.* Retrieved from http://www.cdc.gov/nchhstp/socialdeterminants/faq.html

Chamorro, R., & Flores-Ortiz, Y. (2000). Acculturation and disordered eating patterns among Mexican American women. *International Journal of Eating Disorders, 28*(1), 125–129. doi:10.1002/(SICI)1098-108X(200007)28:1<125::AID- EAT16>3.0.CO;2-9

Clarke, L. H. (2002). Older women's perceptions of ideal body weights: The tensions between health and appearance motivations for weight loss. *Ageing and Society, 22*(6), 751–773. doi:10.1017/S0144686X02008905

Corrigan, P. W., & Kleinlein, P. (2004). The impact of mental illness stigma. In P. W. Corrigan (Ed.), *On the stigma of mental illness: Practical strategies for research and social change.* Washington, DC: American Psychological Association.

Crawford, R. (1980). Healthism and the medicalization of everyday life. *International Journal of Health Services, 10*(3), 365–388. doi:10.2190/3H2H-3XJN-3KAY-G9NY

Crenshaw, K. (1989). Demarginalizing the intersection of race and sex: A black feminist critique of antidiscrimination doctrine, feminist theory, and antiracist politics. *The University of Chicago Legal Forum, 140*, 139–167. Retrieved from http://0 heinonline.org.libcat.widener.edu/HOL/Page?public=false&handle=hein.journals/uchclf1989&id=143

Danford, D. E., & Huber, A. M. (1981). Eating dysfunctions in an institutionalized mentally retarded population. *Appetite: Journal for Intake Research, 2*(4), 281–292. doi:10.1016/S0195-6663(81)80017-7

de Zwaan, M. (2001). Binge eating disorder and obesity. *International Journal of Obesity and Related Metabolic Disorders, 25*(Suppl 1), S51–S55. Retrieved from http://eds.b.ebscohost.com/eds/detail/detail?sid=4ba363e6-3302-4622-80c3

ec414b441f25%40sessionmgr107&vid=0&hid=112&bdata=
JnNpdGU9ZWRzLWxpdmU%3d#AN=9384165&db=aph

Dolan, B. (1989). Cross-cultural aspects of anorexia nervosa and bulimia: A review. *International Journal of Eating Disorders, 10*(1), 67–78. doi:10.1002/1098 108X(199101)10:1<67::AID-EAT2260100108>3.0.CO;2-N

Donini, L. M., Savina, C., & Cannella, C. (2003). Eating habits and appetite control in the elderly: The anorexia of aging. *International Psychogeriatrics, 15*(1), 73–87. doi:10.1017/S1041610203008779

Felstrom, A., Mulryan, N., Reidy, M., & Hillery, J. (2005). Refining diagnoses: Applying the DC-LD to an Irish population with intellectual disability. *Journal of Intellectual Disability Research, 49*(11), 813–819. Retrieved from http://www.ncbi.nlm.nih.gov/pubmed/16207278

Fernández-Aranda, F., Pinheiro, A. P., Tozzi, F., Thornton, L. M., Fichter, M. M., Halmi, K. A.,…Bulik, C. M. (2007). Symptom profile of major depressive disorder in women with eating disorders. *Australian and New Zealand Journal of Psychiatry, 41*(1), 24–31. Retrieved from http://www.ncbi.nlm.nih.gov/pubmed/17464678

Gard, M. C. E., & Freeman, C. P. (1995). The dismantling of a myth: A review of eating disorders and socioeconomic status. *International Journal of Eating Disorders, 20*(1), 1–12. doi:10.1002/(SICI)1098-108X(199607)20:1<1::AID-EAT1>3.0.CO;2-M

Garner, D. M. (1997, January). The 1997 body image survey results. *Psychology Today, 30*, 30.

Gerber, L. (2011). *Seeking the straight and narrow: Weight loss and sexual reorientation in evangelical America.* Chicago, IL: University of Chicago Press.

Godart, N. T., Berthoz, S., Rein, Z., Perdereau, F., Lang, F., & Venisse, J. L. (2006). Does the frequency of anxiety and depressive disorders differ between diagnostic subtypes of anorexia nervosa and bulimia? *International Journal of Eating Disorders, 39*(8), 772–778. Retrieved from http://www.ncbi.nlm.nih.gov/pubmed/16721840

Godart, N. T., Perdereau, F., Rein, Z., Berthoz, S., Wallier, J., Jeammet, P., & Flament, M. F. (2007). Comorbidity studies of eating disorders and mood disorders: Critical review of the literature. *Journal of Affective Disorders, 97*(1–3), 37–49. doi:10.1016/j.jad.2006.06.023

Gravestock, S. (2000). Review: Eating disorders in adults with intellectual disability. *Journal of Intellectual Disability Research, 44*(6), 625–637. doi:10.1046/j.1365-2788.2000.00308.x

Gross, S. M., Ireys, H. T., & Kinsman, S. L. (2000). Young women with physical disabilities: Risk factors for symptoms of eating disorders. *Journal of Developmental and Behavioral Pediatrics, 21*(2), 87–96. Retrieved from http://www.ncbi.nlm.nih.gov/pubmed/10791476

Hall, C. C. I. (1995). Asian eyes: Body image and eating disorders of Asian and Asian American women. *Eating Disorders: The Journal of Treatment and Prevention, 3*(1), 8–19. doi:10.1080/10640269508249141

Hove, O. (2004). Weight survey on adults with mental retardation living in the community. *Research in Developmental Disabilities, 25*(1), 9–17. doi:10.1016/j.ridd.2003.04.004

Hove, O. (2007). Survey on dysfunctional eating behavior in adult persons with intellectual disability living in the community. *Research in Development Disabilities, 28*(1), 1–8. doi:10.1016/j.ridd.2006.10.004

Hudson, J. I., Hiripi, E., Pope, H. G., Jr., & Kessler, R. C. (2007). The prevalence and correlates of eating disorders in the National Comorbidity Survey replication. *Biological Psychiatry, 61*(1), 348–358. doi:10.1016/j.biopsych.2006.03.040

Iancu, I., Spivak, B., Ratzoni, G., Apter, A., & Weizman, A. (1994). The sociocultural theory in the development of anorexia nervosa. *Psychopathology, 27*(1/2), 29–36. doi:10.1159/000284845

Jane, D. M., Hunter, G. C., & Lozzi, B. M. (1999). Do Cuban American women suffer from eating disorders? Effects of media exposure and acculturation. *Hispanic Journal of Behavioral Sciences, 21*(2), 212–218. doi:10.1177/0739986399212007

Jones, C. J., & Samuel, J. (2010). The diagnosis of eating disorders in adults with learning disabilities: Conceptualization and implications for clinical practice. *European Eating Disorders Review, 18*(5), 352–366. doi:10.1002/erv.1007

Kempa, M. L., & Thomas, A. J. (2000). Culturally sensitive assessment and treatment of eating disorders. *Eating Disorders: The Journal of Treatment and Prevention, 8*(1), 17–30. doi:10.1080/10640260008251209

Kilpatrick, M., Ohannessian, C., & Bartholomew, J. B. (1999). Adolescent weight management and perceptions: An analysis of the National Longitudinal Study of Adolescent Health. *Journal of School Health, 69*(4), 148–152. doi:10.1111/j.1746-1561.1999.tb04173.x

Kuh, D. (2007). A life course approach to healthy aging, frailty, and capability. *Journal of Gerontology, Biological Sciences and Medical Sciences, 62*(7), 717–721. doi:10.1093/gerona/62.7.717

Lake, A. J., Staiger, P. K., & Glowinski, H. (2000). Effect of Western culture on women's attitudes to eating and perceptions of body shape. *International Journal of Eating Disorders, 27*(1), 83–89. doi:10.1002/(SICI)1098-108X(200001)27:13.0.CO;2-J

Landi, F., Onder, G., Gambassi, G., Perdone, C., Carbonin, P., & Bernabei, R. (2000). Body mass index and mortality among hospitalized patients. *Archive of Internal Medicine, 160*(17), 2641–2644. doi:10.1001/archinte.160.17.2641

Landi, F., Russo, A., Liperoti, R., Tosato, M., Barillaro, C., Pahor, M.,...Onder, G. (2010). Anorexia, physical function, and incident disability among the frail elderly population: Results from the ilSIRENTE study. *Journal of the American Medical Directors Association, 11*(4), 268–274. doi:10.1016/j.jamda.2009.12.088

Lavender, J. M., Wonderlich, S. A., Crosby, R. D., Engel, S. G., Mitchell, J. E., Crow, S. J.,...Le Grange, D. (2013). Personality-based subtypes of anorexia nervosa: Examining validity and utility using baseline clinical variables and ecological momentary assessment. *Behavioral Research and Therapy, 51*(8), 512–517. doi:10.1016/j.brat.2013.05.007

Lebow, J., Sim, L. A., & Kransdorf, L. N. (2015). Prevalence of a history of overweight and obesity in adolescents with restrictive eating disorders. *Journal of Adolescent Health, 56*(1), 19–24. doi:10.1016/j.jadohealth.2014.06.005

Macpherson-Sánchez, AE. (2015). Integrating fundamental concepts of obesity and eating disorders: Implications for the obesity epidemic. *American Journal of Public Health, 105*(4), e71–e85.

Maine, M., & Kelly, J. (2005). *The body myth: Adult women and the pressure to be perfect.* Hoboken, NJ: John Wiley & Sons, Inc.

Maresh, R. D., & Willard, S. G. (1996). Anorexia nervosa in an African-American female of a lower socioeconomic background. *European Eating Disorders Review, 4*(2), 95–99. doi:10.1002/ (SICI)1099-0968(199606)4:2<95::AID-ERV149>3.0.CO;2-P

Martone, A. M., Onder, G., Vetrano, D. L., Ortolani, E., Tosato, M., Marzetti, E., & Landi, F. (2013). Anorexia of aging: A modifiable risk factor for fragility. *Nutrients, 5*(1), 4126–4133. doi:10.3390/nu5104126

Miller, A. (2014). Losing weight, but not healthy. *Monitor on Psychology, 45*(11), 54. Retrieved from http://www.apa.org/monitor/2014/12/losing-weight.aspx

Morley, J. E. (1997). Anorexia of aging: Physiologic and pathologic. *American Journal of Clinical Nutrition, 66*(4), 760–773. Retrieved from http://www.ncbi. nlm.nih.gov/pubmed/9322549

Morley, J. E. (2007). Weight loss in the nursing home. *Journal of the American Medical Directors Association, 8*(4), 201–204. Retrieved from http://www.ncbi. nlm.nih.gov/pubmed/17498601

Müller, A., Claes, L., Mitchell, J. E., Fischer, J., Horbach, T., & de Zwaan, M. (2012). Binge eating and temperament in morbidly obese prebariatric surgery patients. *European Eating Disorders Review, 20*(1), 91–95. doi:10.1002/erv.1126

National Eating Disorders Association. (2015a). *Eating disorders in women of color: Explanations and implications.* Retrieved from http://www.nationaleatingdisorders.org/ eating-disorders-women-color-explanations-and-implications

National Eating Disorders Association. (2015b). *What's age got to do with it?* Retrieved from http://www.nationaleatingdisorders.org/whats-age-got-do-it

National Eating Disorders Association. (2015c). *Size diversity.* Retrieved from http://www.nationaleatingdisorders.org/size-diversity

Neumark-Sztainer, D., Story, M., Hannan, P. J., Perry, C. L., & Irving, L. M. (2002). Weight-related concerns and behaviors among overweight and nonoverweight adolescents: Implications for preventing weight-related disorders. *Archive of Pediatric and Adolescent Medicine, 156*(2), 171–178. doi:10.1001/ archpedi.156.2.171

Neumark-Sztainer, D., Story, M., Resnick, M. D., & Blum, R. W. (1998). Lessons learned about adolescent nutrition from the Minnesota Adolescent Health Survey. *Journal of American Dietic Association, 98*(12), 1449–1456. doi:10.1016/ S0002-8223(98)00329-0

Oliver, M. (1983). *Social work with disabled people.* Basingstoke, UK: Macmillan.

Osvald, L. L., & Sodowsky, G. R. (1993). Eating disorders of white American, racial and ethnic minority American, and international women. *Journal of Multicultural Counseling and Development, 21*(3), 143–154. doi:10.1002/j.2161-1912.1993.tb00594.x

Ottati, V., Bodenhausen, G. V., & Newman, L. S. (2004). Social psychological models of mental illness stigma. In P. W. Corrigan (Ed.), *On the stigma of mental illness: Practical strategies for research and social change.* Washington, DC: American Psychological Association.

Patton, G. C., Wood, K., & Johnson-Sabine, E. (1986). Physical illness: A risk factor in anorexia nervosa. *The British Journal of Psychiatry, 149*(6), 756–759. doi:10.1192/bjp.149.6.756

Peters, S. (1996). The politics of disabled identity. In L. Barton (Ed.), *Disability and society: Emerging issues and insight.* London, UK: Longman.

Phinney, J. S. (1989). Stages of ethnic identity development in minority group adolescents. *Journal of Early Adolescence, 9*(1/2), 34–49. doi:10.1177/0272431689091004

Pinquart, M. (2012). Self-esteem of children and adolescents with chronic illness: A meta-analysis. *Child: Care, Health, and Development, 39*(2), 153–161. doi:10.1111/j.1365-2214.2012.01397.x

Puhl, R. M., Moss-Racusin, C. A., & Schwartz, M. B. (2007). Internalization of weight bias: Implications for binge eating and emotional well-being. *Obesity, 15*(1), 19–23. Retrieved from http://www.ncbi.nlm.nih.gov/pubmed/17228027

Quick, V. M., Byrd-Bredbenner, C., & Neumark-Sztainer, D. (2013). Chronic illness and disordered eating: A discussion of the literature. *Advances in Nutrition, 4*(3), 277–286. doi:10.3945/an.112.003608

Reynaert, C., Zdanowicz, N., Janne, P., & Jacques, D. (2010). Depression and sexuality. *Psychiatrica Danubina, 22*(S1), 111–113. Retrieved from http://www.hdbp.org/psychiatria_danubina/pdf/dnb_vol22_sup/dnb_vol22_sup_111.pdf

Robinson, T. B., Killen, J. D., Litt, I. F., Hammer, L. D., Wilson, D. M., Haydel, K. F.,... Taylor, C. B. (1996). Ethnicity and body dissatisfaction: Are Hispanic and Asian girls at increased risk for eating disorders? *Journal of Adolescent Health, 19*(6), 384–393. Retrieved from http://www.ncbi.nlm.nih.gov/pubmed/8969369

Rogers, L., Resnick, M. D., Mitchell, J. E., & Blum, R. W. (1997). The relationship between socioeconomic status and eating-disordered behaviors in a community sample of adolescent girls. *International Journal of Eating Disorders, 22*(1), 15–23. Retrieved from http://www.ncbi.nlm.nih.gov/pubmed/9140731

Shisslak, C.M., Crago, M., & Estes, L.S. (1995). The spectrum of eating disturbances. *International Journal of Eating Disorders, 18*(3), 209–219. doi:10.1002/1098 108X(199511)18:33.0.CO;2-E

Sim, L. A., Lebow, J., & Billings, M. (2013). Eating disorders in adolescents with a history of obesity. *Pediatrics, 132*(4), e1026–e1030. doi:10.1542/peds.2012-3940

Smith, F. M., Latchford, G. J., Hall, R. M., & Dickson, R. A. (2008). Do chronic medical conditions increase the risk of eating disorder? A cross-sectional investigation of eating pathology in adolescents females with scoliosis and diabetes. *Journal of Adolescent Health, 42*(1), 58–63. doi:10.1016/j.jadohealth.2007.08.008

Soenen, S., & Chapman, I. M. (2013). Body weight, anorexia, and undernutrition in older people. *Journal of the American Medical Directors Association, 14*(9), 642–648. doi:10.1016/j.jamda.2013.02.004

Spitzer, B. L., Henderson, K. A., & Zivian, M. T. (1999). Gender differences in population versus media body sizes: A comparison over four decades. *Sex Roles, 40*(7), 545–565. doi:10.1023/A:1018836029738

Story, M., French, S. A., Resnick, M. D., & Blum, R. W. (1995). Ethnic/racial and socioeconomic differences in dieting behaviors and body image perceptions in adolescents. *International Journal of Eating Disorders, 18*(2), 173–181. doi:10.1002/1098-108X(199509)18:2<173::AID-EAT2260180210>3.0.CO;2-Q

Tareen, A., Hodes, M., & Rangel, L. (2005). Non-fat-phobic anorexia nervosa in British South Asian adolescents. *International Journal of Eating Disorders, 37*(2), 161–165. doi:10.1002/eat.20080

Thompson, B. W. (1994). *A hunger so wide and so deep: A multiracial view of women's eating problems.* Minneapolis, MN: University of Minnesota Press.

Tierney, S. (2001). A reluctance to be defined 'disabled': How can the social model of disability enhance understanding of anorexia? *Disability and Society, 16*(5), 749–764. doi:10.1080/09687590120070105

Vartanian, L. R., & Smyth, J. M. (2013). Primum non nocere: Obesity stigma and public health. *Journal of Bioethical Inquiry, 10*(1), 49–57. doi:10.1007/s11673-012-9412-9

Villarejo, C., Jiménez-Murcia, S., Álvarez-Moya, E., Granero, R., Penelo, E., Treasure, J.,…Vilarrasa, N. (2014). Loss of control over eating: A description of the eating disorder/obesity spectrum in women. *European Eating Disorders Review, 22*(1), 25–31. doi:10.1002/erv.2267

Visvanathan, R. (2015). Anorexia of aging. *Clinical Geriatric Medicine, 31*(3), 417–427. doi:10.1016/j.cger.2015.04.012

Wade, T. D., Keski-Rahkonen, A., & Hudson, J. (2011). Epidemiology of eating disorders. In M. Tsuang & M. Tohen (Eds.), *Textbook in psychiatric epidemiology* (3rd ed., pp. 343–360). New York, NY: Wiley.

Watkins, B., Sutton, V., & Lask, B. (2001). Is physical illness a risk factor for eating disorders in children and adolescents? A preliminary investigation. *Eating Behavior, 2*(3), 209–214. doi:10.1016/S1471-0153(01)00029-0

Wolf, N. (2002). *The beauty myth: How images of beauty are used against women* (2nd ed.). New York, NY: Harper Perennial.

Wonderlich, S. A., Lilenfeld, L. R., Riso, L. P., Engel, S., & Mitchell, J. E. (2005). Personality and anorexia nervosa. *International Journal of Eating Disorders, 37*(S1), S68–S71. doi:10.1002/eat.20120

World Health Organization. (2016). *Social determinants of health.* Retrieved from http://www.who.int/social_determinants/sdh_definition/en/

What Is Sexuality, Anyway?

Chapter 3

Before we can dive into the ways in which women with anorexia experience sexuality, we need to get clear on what I mean when I say *sexuality* in the first place. Because for most people, it's not at all what they imagine, which often falls into the realm of sexual behavior or identity. I've spent years of my life as a student of Human Sexuality Studies and as a sex researcher, trying to explain the vastness – the complexity – of sexuality to people. This is the hill I will die on.

When people realize what I do, they often ask me, "You study sex? What does that mean?" Or, jokingly, "What is there to know?" First of all, if you think that understanding (or even *having*) sex is as simple as putting the right-shaped peg into the right-shaped hole, you're probably having absolutely terrible sex. But moreover, would you ever ask something like that of a physicist? As if gravity can be simplified into "what goes up must come down," as if your very basic understanding of a concept is comparable to an expert's?

And for folks who *don't* think of intercourse as soon as the S-word comes out of my mouth, they usually think I'm referring to orientation or identity and that I study the LGBTQIA+ (lesbian, gay, bisexual, transgender, queer, intersex, asexual, and more sexual minorities) spectrum. But nope. It's not that either.

Not *entirely*, anyway.

Yes, sexuality is an overarching concept that includes orientation and identity, as well as the aforementioned sexual behavior, but that's not where it ends. That's not even where it starts. Sexuality is a phenomenon that encompasses various biological, psychological, and sociocultural factors, and that shows up for everyone differently, in both slight and astounding ways. It's an expression of different parts of who we are as individual people and collective groups, a complicated web of identities and experiences that interact to create realities as simultaneously unique and common as a fingerprint. Sexuality encompasses body image, pleasure, love, vulnerability, gender, orientation, reproduction, anatomy, and even acts of violence, such as rape and incest. And even *that's* not all!

Luckily, there's a model to help make sense of this vast interconnectedness in a simple, visual way.

THE CIRCLES OF SEXUALITY

This model is one of my favorites.

You know that feeling when you have an epiphany, where something that you always knew to be true, deep down, is suddenly presented to you in a word or a visual? It's like when I first heard the word *bisexual* in the eighth grade and finally understood the confusion I'd felt my whole life, being gray in a category I'd thought could only be black or white. That's sort of what this model is like for me. It's less life-changing than the validation of the existence of bisexuality, but it's still exciting.

The Circles of Sexuality is a model that was created by Dr. Dennis Dailey in 1981, originally as a tool to explore the complex dynamics of sexual expression and aging. But the model has since been adapted, modified, and broadened, perhaps most notably by Advocates for Youth, which is a Washington, DC-based organization helping young people make informed choices around sexual health. And the model has become a useful way to understand sexuality as a complex intersection of experiences, as well as a diverse and interdisciplinary field.

What Is Sexuality, Anyway?

Personally, I love this model because it's useful in helping people consider sexuality in broader terms, rather than simply the experience of sexual desire, arousal, and intercourse. According to Advocates for Youth (2018, para. 1), in this model, sexuality is inclusive of "all the feelings, thoughts, and behaviors associated with [gender], being attractive and being in love, as well as being in relationships that include sexual intimacy and sensual and sexual activity."

All the feelings, thoughts, and behaviors!

I know that sounds like a lot – and it is! – but the Circles of Sexuality model provides a neat and concise way to exemplify that. Let me show you:

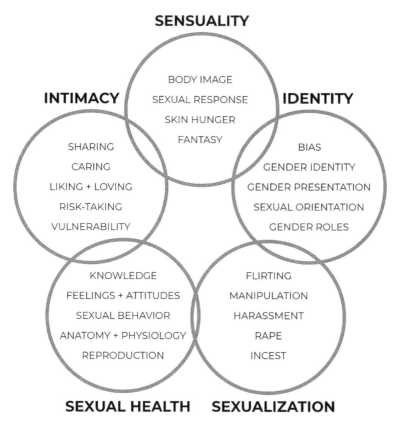

Figure 3.1 The Circles of Sexuality model illustrates the complexity and overlapping nature of sexuality.

What you're looking at is an illustrated representation of the model, one that I adapted from Dailey's 1981 original. It shows five circles that each represent a broad category of sexuality: sensuality, intimacy, identity, sexual health, and sexualization. Within each circle are more focused categories of sexual experience that are encapsulated within that circle. For example, within *Sensuality*, you also see skin hunger and fantasy. These smaller categories help make up the larger, overarching category.

The cool thing is that the circles overlap – which indicates that all of the experiences listed are related to and can affect one another. That means not only that sexuality encompasses a whole lot, but that it can also get really complicated.

And it's in using this model that I'm going to break down the relationship between anorexia nervosa and women's sexuality. Because it allows for the individual pieces that make up a person's sexuality to be explored both separately and in-depth, while acknowledging how these small pieces interact with one another. This is especially important because as we talk about various aspects of sexuality for women with anorexia, you'll notice that there are a lot of caveats like, "But *x* might affect *y*, which might be affected by *z*, so who the hell knows what the story is here?" If you're a researcher, you're used to this way of thinking. We draw conclusions based on syllogisms (i.e., "This is true, and this is true, so probably this combined thing is true"). But we also need to name the mediating factors that might interrupt the truth we think we've found.

And I think that this understanding of sexuality as vast and complex is important, as it more clearly addresses the intricacies of a person's experience with various aspects of their sexuality.

Now that we understand that sexuality is complicated and that it involves a lot more than we all probably originally thought, we can move through each circle, taking a tour of the various ways in which women with anorexia tend to experience different aspects of their sexuality.

This book is set up the same way that my dissertation was: Using the Circles of Sexuality as a guide for how to break down information, we will go through all of the research that I've found on how women with anorexia experience sexuality. That means that you can read this in a few ways: You can read it front to back, beginning to end. Or you can skip to the sections that are of most interest to you, and then backtrack if you feel like it. There is no right or wrong here. You can decide how it's of most use to you.

My hope is that you come out the other side of this book with a broader understanding of sexuality as a concept, a more in-depth comprehension of how sexuality and anorexia interact, and a meaningful sense of validation for your own experiences or observations. However you go about meeting those ends works for me.

REFERENCES

Advocates for Youth. (2018). *An explanation of the circles of sexuality.* Retrieved from http://www.advocatesforyouth.org/for-professionals/lesson-plans professionals/200

Dailey, D. (1981). Sexual expression and aging. In F. Berghorn & D. Schafer (Eds.), *The dynamics of aging: Original essays on the processes and experiences of growing old* (pp. 311–330). Boulder, CO: Westview Press.

Sexual Health

Chapter 4

Ah, yes. The birds and the bees.

Most people, when I tell them that I'm a sex writer, researcher, and educator, envision this circle: me, at an old-school chalkboard, with diagrams of uterine anatomy and flowcharts of menstrual cycles. They picture young kids moving through puberty, giggling at the word *penis*.

And yes. This would be an accurate depiction of many sex education classes – the ones that don't try to scare the shit out of you with way-blown-out-of-proportion warnings about sexually transmitted infections, anyway.

So let's start here – at everyone's favorite memories of watching live births and learning to roll a condom down a banana.

According to Advocates for Youth (2018, para. 22), this circle refers to a person's "capacity to reproduce and the behaviors and attitudes that make sexual relationships healthy and enjoyable." Here, we're talking about factual information about reproduction, feelings and attitudes toward sexual expression, various forms of sexual behavior, reproductive and sexual anatomy and physiology, and sexual reproduction. We're talking about what we know, think, and do related to the physical, biological experience of sexual activity.

We're talking about the technical stuff here.

And it's actually what we learn within these pages that sets the stage for my entire dissertation process. Thinking about how women with anorexia experience sexuality on this very basic level is what got the wheels in my brain turning, trying to sort out what was missing from the conversation.

And in fact, because most folks' first thought when it comes to sexuality is *exactly this kind of stuff*, you may have bought this book specifically to learn more about this circle. As such, it's the perfect place to start.

FEELINGS AND ATTITUDES

We all have feelings and attitudes – values, even – when it comes to thinking about sex. In fact, during my Master's program, I had to go through a desensitization process called Sexual Attitude Reassessment (SAR) seminars. The point of an SAR is to force us to think long and hard about our feelings and attitudes toward various aspects of sexuality so that we can unpack them and take some of the subjectivity away. After all, if I'm working as a sex therapist, for instance, and I have incredibly strong negative feelings against, say, polyamory or foot paraphilia, I could inadvertently really hurt a client with my reaction to their telling me they're into it! SARs help you understand what you think and feel, and they challenge you to restructure your thinking to a more neutral place.

When it comes to women with anorexia, there is strong evidence to show common feelings of aversion, avoidance, and immaturity toward sex – and this leads to the supposition that this population is more likely to avoid sexual activity at higher rates (Gonidakis, Kravvariti, Fabello, & Varsou, 2016).

Even clinicians who work with eating disorder clients describe their clients' personalities in ways that relate to sexuality. One study showed that clinicians described their clients with restrictive anorexia as exerting more control and having more constrained personalities, sometimes using words like *childlike, prim,* and *proper* to describe them (Eddy, Novotny, & Westen, 2004). All-in-all, researchers found that these personality types were predictive of a more immature sexuality. Similarly, other research has shown that in conversations with women with anorexia, they frequently report a lack of interest in – or even show a disgust with – sex (Pinheiro et al., 2010; Ruuska, Kaltiala-Heino, Koivisto, & Rantanen, 2003).

In my own research, I generally found these ideas reproduced: My participants tended toward being disinterested in or apathetic toward sex, with some also being actively averse to it. "I guess I just don't think about it that much," Gail explained, highlighting the most common reaction that I heard. "I could've taken it or left it."

This attitude – that sex is unimportant, not necessarily hated or avoided, but certainly not compelling – was frequently expressed by my participants. Winnie told me that because she has trouble understanding why one would want to engage in sexual activity, "I definitely describe myself as, like, an eleven-year-old."

One-quarter of my participants specifically expressed a strong distaste for, disgust with, or fear of sex. They named feelings such as panic, fear, guilt, anger, and shame as associated with the act for them. For these participants, dissociation tended to be a common coping mechanism for avoiding the psychological experience of sexual activity. "When I have sexual experiences, I'm generally very disconnected from my body," Rachel said, "and so I'm not entirely present, mentally or physically, in those experiences."

Olivia explained her thought process when she's engaging in sex thusly: "When is this going to be over? How much longer is this going to last?" She said, "I just feel kind of gross. [I] can't shower quick enough."

Of course, what's tricky here is the-chicken-or-the-egg paradox: Which comes first? If women with anorexia tend to be more controlling and restrictive in every aspect of their lives, it could simply be these same personality traits that lead to *both* the eating disorder *and* the relative disinterest in sex. Their disinterest in or disgust with sex might have nothing to do with the eating disorder in and of itself, but rather, a mediating factor, such as personality.

Eating disorders may be related to crises of sexual identity – that is, they may affect sexual development – in young women (Romejko-Borowiec, 2004). In general, women with eating disorders are more ambivalent, overall, toward sex – and tellingly, the more invested they are in their body image, the less interest they have in sex.

As diagnostic criteria for anorexia include a preoccupation with body image (American Psychiatric Association, 2013a), you may be thinking, "Wait! Could this affect women with anorexia in particular?" And the answer is yes. Women with anorexia aren't only more avoidant of sex, but also more *content* with that avoidance, as compared to women with other eating disorders (Romejko-Borowiec, 2004). That is, they're cool with the fact that they aren't engaging in sexual activity; they don't crave or desire it. They don't necessarily see it as problematic for them; it's just a fact of their lives.

In my own research, participants expressed similar experiences. Cali explained, "[Sex] is not something that's missing from my life. It's just absent." She went on, "It doesn't register as something that I want or need or would make my life significantly better in any way. It's not something that I miss or…want for."

Eleana's experience was similar: "I don't have any need for [sex]… It's like whatever. It doesn't bother me."

Even two years into recovery, women with anorexia have been found to be significantly less likely than women with bulimia to report even having masturbated in that time (Morgan, Wiederman, & Pryor, 1995), which could suggest that the eating disorder itself is less relevant than women's personalities.

But research also shows that weight and diet restoration – that is, recovery, especially for women who are underweight due to their eating disorder – is linked to an increased sex drive in women with eating disorders (Morgan, Reid, & Lacey, 1999).

Corroborating this research, approximately two-thirds of my participants named that they find themselves *less* interested in sex when their eating disorder is active and/or *more* interested in sex during bouts of recovery. "As far as...sex drive, when I'm in my eating disorder, it's absolutely zero," Rachel explained. And Kaylee noted, "Since I've been in recovery, I have felt much more of a sex drive than I've ever had before, which is kind of a surprise."

Perhaps significantly, four of my participants actively identified as asexual. And three of them described themselves as having very high sex drives, sometimes to the point of compulsion. Two of those participants experience the binge/purge subtype of anorexia, which could be significant, as women with bulimia, an eating disorder also associated with cycles of bingeing and purging, tend to describe their relationship to sex similarly (Eddy et al., 2004; Morgan et al., 1995).

Does this mean, automatically, that a woman with anorexia is bound to hate sex? No. But it might suggest that the personality traits associated with women who develop anorexia may also be linked to a disinterest in sex.

PUBERTY

Looking back on it, puberty is a relatively terrifying time – especially when the trusted adults in your life, like your parents or teachers, for instance, don't do nearly enough to prepare you for the phenomenon.

Hair starts growing in new places. For many of us with ovaries – and therefore, a likely abundance of estrogen – our hips, thighs, butts, and breasts expand so quickly, we get stretch marks. And some of us with uteruses wake up one morning to find blood pooling between our legs. Fun times!

And the feelings and attitudes toward sexuality that we just discussed make a lot of sense within a larger context exploring the potential relationship between the onset of puberty and the development of anorexia in women.

When I spoke with my participants about their experiences with body image, several common themes emerged, including this one: While many named that their body image had been negative since childhood, more pointed to puberty and adolescence as significant turning points for their relationships with their bodies – and therefore, food.

Siobhan hit the nail on the head: "I just saw that I was becoming a woman…and that meant I had body changes." More specifically, Gail described, "Along the way somewhere, I kind of started thinking…not even consciously…that I'm taking up too much space."

Gina noted that, for her, the experience of "going into sixth grade and just basically being metaphorically slaughtered," particularly as a "bigger girl," affected her psychologically, at a time when self-concept is already fragile.

The experience of puberty, along with the associated hormonal changes, has been associated with higher body dissatisfaction and decreased self-esteem in young women, research suggests (Klump, 2013).

And of course it is. Young women are trying to cope with their changing shapes, especially when many of their peers still have prepubescent bodies (Ruuska, Kaltiala-Heino, Rantanen, & Koivisto, 2005). When we think about the fact that we live in a cultural climate where svelte, androgynous female bodies have been revered in modeling and media in the latter half of the 20th century, it makes sense that young cisgender women with a predisposition for eating disorder development might be triggered by the experience of puberty.

That early onset puberty may be a risk factor in eating disorder development, especially for bulimia (Ruuska et al., 2003), might feel like a no-brainer!

Specifically, it might be young women's *attitudes* toward puberty that are more significant predictive factors of eating disorder development than the biological experience itself – and women with eating disorders have more significantly negative attitudes toward puberty than unaffected women (Mangweth-Matzek, Rupp, Hausmann, Kemmler, & Biebl, 2007).

A 2016 study that I co-authored notes that, for adolescent women with anorexia, "starvation and weight loss have been nothing more than a frantic effort to postpone, or even inhibit, the terrorizing welcoming of sexual maturation and intimate relationships" (Gonidakis et al., 2016, p. 20).

Terrorizing.

That's one way to describe puberty, alright.

Some women find that their relationships to their bodies have always been complicated; in my own study, Winnie told me, "I've always felt like [my body] needed to be altered and edited and shrunk in order to be acceptable, manageable." But it makes sense that for many more, the sudden changes that come with puberty can be triggering.

SEXUAL BEHAVIOR

Unsurprisingly, these negative attitudes toward sexuality, as well as overall physical and emotional sexual immaturity, might be associated with decreased sexual behavior in women with anorexia. Go figure.

It's important to note, though, that sexual behavior doesn't only include intercourse – the first thing we tend to think of in our allosexual, cisheteronormative, phallocentric society. Sexual behavior includes *all* kinds of activities, from kissing and making out to manual and oral sex, and more. Different people experience sexuality differently, and allowing folks to define "sexual behavior" for themselves is paramount.

Women with eating disorders are less likely to have experienced sexual intercourse and to be engaged in sexual relationships, overall, compared with unaffected women (Romejko-Borowiec, 2004). However, even compared to women with bulimia, women with anorexia have fewer sexual experiences. Women with bulimia are more likely to engage in a variety of sexual activities – including masturbation, intercourse, and fantasy – than women with anorexia (Wiederman, Pryor, & Morgan, 1996). Women with bulimia have also been noted to be more likely, overall, to engage in more frequent sexual activity with more partners than women with anorexia (Wiederman et al., 1996), something that could be related, again, to personality types associated with these two illnesses.

However, women with anorexia have reported engaging in sexual activity for the sole purpose of feeling connected to or pleasing their partners, even when it doesn't result in their own enjoyment or satisfaction (Newton, Boblin, Brown, &

Ciliska, 2005, 2006). On the one hand, this is a red flag: No one should feel coerced or manipulated into sex, even implicitly by social expectations. On the other, it's necessary to acknowledge that there are several drives toward sexual behavior, and one's own personal pleasure or satisfaction isn't the only reason why people engage in sex.

Within eating disorder research, there is a significant amount of literature discussing the relationship between anorexia and sexual functioning specifically. Sexual functioning is essentially a person's ability (or not) to experience pleasure, desire, arousal, and orgasm. When folks don't experience these things in a way that feels normative (which, of course, is a fluid concept), and if it causes them distress, we call that *sexual dysfunction*.

Personally, I think that's an intense label to throw on someone who simply experiences their body differently, and there are a lot of critiques to be made about the ways in which researchers have conceptualized female sexual dysfunction. Namely, researchers, such as Masters and Johnson – who have become household names again, thanks to the Showtime series *Masters of Sex* – labeled cisgender women's experiences as quote-unquote "dysfunctional" if they didn't match cisgender men's experiences. That is, they let cisgender men be the prototype for normalcy, and they measured cisgender women against that. Newsflash: Our bodies work differently. And thus, the very concept of (dys)functionality can be questioned – and has been, most notably in Shere Hite's 1976 *Hite Report on Female Sexuality*.

In 1991, researchers conducted a study on self-assessed conceptualizations of sexual functioning in women with eating disorders – that is, how women with eating disorders understand their own experience of sexuality (Rothschild, Fagan, Woodall, & Andersen, 1991). They found that while women with eating disorders, compared to one another, appear "to be relatively homogeneous regarding sexual functioning" (p. 391), women with eating disorders have very low sexual functioning and satisfaction compared to unaffected women. The researchers noted that "[a]s a group, the patients described the frequencies of intercourse, masturbation, kissing, petting, and sexual fantasies at approximately the 20th percentile" of unaffected women (p. 391).

That's a pretty big difference!

Of course, this 1991 study is outdated, especially because it was done using *DSM-III* criteria; this is true for a lot of the research done pre-*DSM-V*, which explains why so much of this conversation centers on comparing anorexia and bulimia, leaving out the newly diagnosable binge eating disorder. However, more recent studies also confirm that women with eating disorders experience lower sexual functioning and satisfaction than unaffected women: A 2016 review of the literature found that all of the included studies showed a negative relationship between anorexia and sexual attitudes and functioning (Gonidakis et al., 2016).

There are many potential mediating factors for this relationship, however, some of which will be discussed in this book. Depression, sexual violence, personality traits, and body image can be links between women's experience with anorexia and their experience with sexual functioning.

But if *every single recent study* on the subject says that there's a relationship, chances are, there's a relationship.

PREGNANCY

The potential mediating factor of body image comes up a lot when we're talking about the intersection of eating disorders and sexuality. Obviously. If we're talking about women who feel uncomfortable about and in their bodies, it makes sense that they may experience some issues with their sexuality. It's been shown that women with eating disorders are more likely than unaffected women to experience negative body image (Mangweth-Matzek et al., 2007). And in women, negative body image can lead to complications in *all* domains of sexual functioning and satisfaction (La Rocque & Cioe, 2011; Woertman & van den Brink, 2012).

Therefore, it makes sense that whether people with eating disorders experience psychological difficulty with pregnancy, as well as physical complications with conceiving and gestation, has been explored.

What we know is this: Irregularity of menstruation, not eating disorder diagnosis specifically, has been significantly associated with infertility (Maxwell et al., 2011). As amenorrhea – that is, loss of one or more periods – was once considered diagnostic criteria for anorexia, this could associate anorexia diagnoses specifically with difficulty with pregnancy (American Psychiatric Association, 2013b).

And we also know this: Research suggests that fertility and reproductive health issues can be resolved by sustaining recovery for a significant amount of time (Conti, Abraham, & Taylor, 1998; Sullivan, Bulik, Fear, & Pickering, 1998).

The body of a person with severe anorexia (or, more generally, anyone not receiving appropriate caloric intake) shuts down various physiological functions as a way to preserve energy. The incredible amount of energy that it takes to foster another human being's life inside of your body cannot be sustained in a person experiencing malnutrition.

But "because pregnancy is a sensitive time for [those] who struggle" with disordered eating (p. 141), Claire Mysko and Magali Amadeï include a chapter on the issue in their 2009 book *Does This Pregnancy Make Me Look Fat?: The Essential Guide to Loving Your Body Before and After Baby.*

In their book, they discuss a phenomenon dubbed *pregorexia* by the media, which describes the experience of eating disorder symptoms being triggered during pregnancy, in part due to the stress associated with one's changing body. Because body-related anxiety, especially as it pertains to pregnancy, has been socially normalized, pregnant people's concerns about body image and dieting behaviors are often brushed off as normal. Like, "Shrug. Oh well. Join the club." Obstetricians and gynecologists who aren't trained in recognizing the signs of eating disorders often push concerned clients to focus on the health of their growing fetus instead, completely missing the actual issue at hand (Mysko & Amadeï, 2009).

Pregnant people are also often watched closely for "too much" weight gain, pressured to fall within a range of "acceptable" pregnancy weight. It's no wonder that during this time of body stress, folks may develop (sometimes maladaptive) coping mechanisms!

Eating disorders, at the end of the day, are about how we relate to our bodies and how we behave around food. However, they affect much more than that, including our experiences with sex. After all, sexual health is an experience that we have, partly in our bodies. And when one facet of embodiment is thrown off, it can disrupt others.

In the next chapter, we'll talk more about the opposite relationship: not how our eating disorders may relate to our sexuality, but how our sexuality (and more specifically, our histories of trauma) may relate to eating disorder development.

REFERENCES

Advocates for Youth. (2018). *An explanation of the circles of sexuality.* Retrieved from http://www.advocatesforyouth.org/for-professionals/lesson-plans professionals/200

American Psychiatric Association. (2013a). *Diagnostic and statistical manual of mental disorders* (5th ed.). Washington, DC: American Psychiatric Association.

American Psychiatric Association. (2013b). *Feeding and eating disorders fact sheet.* Retrieved from http://www.dsm5.org/documents/eating%20disorders%20fact%20sheet.pdf

Conti, J., Abraham, S., & Taylor, A. (1998). Eating behavior and pregnancy outcome. *Journal of Psychosomatic Research, 44*(3/4), 465–477.

Eddy, K. T., Novotny, C. M., & Westen, D. (2004). Sexuality, personality, and eating disorders. *Eating Disorders, 12*(3), 191–208.

Gonidakis, F., Kravvariti, V., Fabello, M., & Varsou, E. (2016). Anorexia nervosa and sexual function. *Current Sexual Health Reports, 8*(1), 19–26.

Klump, K. L. (2013). Puberty as a critical risk period for eating disorders: A review of human and animal studies. *Hormonal Behavior, 64*(2), 399–410.

La Rocque, C. L., & Cioe, J. (2011). An evaluation of the relationship between body image and sexual avoidance. *Journal of Sex Research, 48*(4), 397–408.

Mangweth-Matzek, B., Rupp, C. I., Hausmann, A., Kemmler, G., & Biebl, W. (2007). Menarche, puberty, and first sexual activities in eating-disordered patients as compared with a psychiatric and a nonpsychiatric control group. *International Journal of Eating Disorders, 40*(8), 705–710.

Maxwell, M., Thornton, L. M., Root, T. L., Pinheiro, A. P., Strober, M., Brandt, H., ... Bulik, C. M. (2011). Life beyond the eating disorder: Education, relationships, and reproduction. *International Journal of Eating Disorders, 44*(3), 225–232.

Morgan, C. D., Wiederman, M. W., & Pryor, T. L. (1995). Sexual functioning and attitudes of eating-disordered women: A follow-up study. *Journal of Sex and Marital Therapy, 21*(2), 67–77.

Morgan, J. D., Reid, F., & Lacey, J. H. (1999). The SCOFF questionnaire: Assessment of a new screening tool for eating disorders. *British Medical Journal, 319*(7223), 1467–1468.

Mysko, C., & Amadeï, M. (2009). *Does this pregnancy make me look fat?: An essential guide to loving your body before and after baby.* Deerfield Beach, FL: Health Communications, Inc.

Newton, M., Boblin, S., Brown, B., & Ciliska, D. (2005). "An engagement-distancing flux": Bringing a voice to experiences with romantic relationships for women with anorexia nervosa. *European Eating Disorders Review, 13*(5), 317–329.

Newton, M., Boblin, S., Brown, B., & Ciliska, D. (2006). Understanding intimacy for women with anorexia nervosa: A phenomenological approach. *European Eating Disorders Review, 14*(1), 43–53.

Pinheiro, A. P., Raney, T. J., Thornton, L. M., Fichter, M. M., Berrettini, W. H., Goldman, D.,...Bulik, C.M. (2010). Sexual functioning in women with eating disorders. *International Journal of Eating Disorders, 43*(2), 123–129.

Romejko-Borowiec, A. (2004). Eating disorders as a specific method of solving the sexual identity crisis. *Archives of Psychiatry and Psychotherapy, 6*(4), 41–48.

Rothschild, B. S., Fagan, P. J., Woodall, C., & Andersen, A. E. (1991). Sexual functioning of female eating-disordered patients. *International Journal of Eating Disorders, 10*(4), 389–394.

Ruuska, J., Kaltiala-Heino, R., Koivisto, A. M., & Rantanen, P. (2003). Puberty, sexual development, and eating disorders in adolescent outpatients. *European Child & Adolescent Psychiatry, 12*(5), 214–220.

Ruuska, J., Kaltiala-Heino, R., Rantanen, P., & Koivisto, A. M. (2005). Psychopathological distress predicts suicidal ideation and self-harm in adolescent eating disorder outpatients. *European Child and Adolescent Psychiatry, 14*(5), 276–281.

Sullivan, P. F., Bulik, C. M., Fear, J. L., & Pickering, A. (1998). Outcome of anorexia nervosa: A case-control study. *American Journal of Psychiatry, 155*(7), 939–946.

Wiederman, M. W., Pryor, T., & Morgan, C. D. (1996). The sexual experience of women diagnosed with anorexia nervosa or bulimia nervosa. *International Journal of Eating Disorders, 19*(2), 109–118.

Woertman, L., & van den Brink, F. (2012). Body image and female sexual functioning and behavior: A review. *Journal of Sex Research, 49*(2/3), 184–211.

Sexualization

Chapter 5

People often think of this circle as the dark side of sexuality. In it, we talk about everything from sexual harassment to sexual assault. And as such, I want to make sure that you're taking care of yourself as you read through this chapter. It isn't easy to talk about the violence that people inflict on others, especially if you or someone close to you has experienced it directly.

As you read this chapter, take it slowly. Recognize when uncomfortable feelings come up for you. Take breaks. Call a friend. If you need or want to, skip this section altogether!

Also know that resources are available to you, should you need them. Contacting your local sexual assault support services organization is one step; you could also call your national hotline. In the United States, the number for RAINN (Rape, Abuse, and Incest National Network) is 1-800-656-4673, and they also have an online chat option at rainn.org.

This circle can be hard to get through, but the reason that we acknowledge and address it is because negative experiences that we have with sexuality can be deeply formative. And when it comes to eating disorders, that's really important – because it can sometimes offer a clue.

In my own research, even without my asking about it outright, more than half of my participants mentioned experiences of abuse in their lives – whether sexual, physical, or emotional; whether in childhood or adulthood. And these participants often talked about these experiences as influential in their psychosexual development.

Of course, we can't assume that anyone with an eating disorder has experienced sexual trauma. And we also can't assume that sexual trauma inevitably leads to an eating disorder. Neither is true. But we *can* say that there are multiple correlations at the intersection of sexualization and eating disorders – and they're worth looking at closely.

OBJECTIFICATION THEORY

To situate ourselves in this chapter, I want to talk a little bit about objectification theory, which was introduced by Fredrickson and Roberts in 1997.

Objectification theory is a framework that explores how womanhood is experienced "in a sociocultural context that sexually objectifies the female body and equates a woman's worth with her body's appearance and sexual functions" and how that affects mental health (Szymanski, Moffitt, & Carr, 2011, p. 6) – that is, how women experience the world, given the effects of oppression at the site of our bodies. Overlapping oppressions (racism, ableism, sizeism, etc.), of course, in addition to sexism, further exacerbate the ways in which women are objectified.

The participants in my research spoke about objectification at length – from multiple lenses of marginalization. One of the themes that emerged in my dissertation was "Sexuality as an Outside Force" – the idea that one-quarter of my participants named sexuality as something separate from themselves, as something that belongs to other people.

"Sexuality has kind of happened to me," Sarika said, referencing her experiences with her marginalized gender, race, and class. "It's like [sexuality] never belongs to you. So trying to find yourself in that is very difficult." She continued, "I felt like I was just trying to navigate what other people dumped on me."

Indeed, participants with multiple marginalized identities – those who were fat, disabled, transgender, of color, and so on – named how their bodies are objectified in the world through intersecting systems of oppression. Adra, at the oppressed intersections of gender, race, and size, said, simply, "I feel like a piece of meat."

Indeed, external objectification – that is, the feeling of being reduced to an object by people in the outside world – is often a violating experience. However, objectification theory also considers internal objectification: the ways in which we internalize harmful messages and apply them to ourselves.

In 2005, for example, one study found that the "internalization of sociocultural standards of beauty mediated the links of sexual objectification experiences to body surveillance, body shame, and eating disorder symptoms" (Moradi, Dirks, & Matteson, 2005, p. 420). That is, the level at which participants subconsciously agreed with social beauty standards impacted how they saw themselves – and how they ate. And it's important to remember that the beauty standard isn't only about being thin – it's also about being white, able, cisgender, and more. The further one is from the social ideal, the more deeply harmful that ideal can be.

A 2012 study explored the experience of self-objectification, defined as the extent to which various body attributes contribute to one's self-concept, in Australian women (Tiggemann & Williams, 2012). They connected self-objectification to a variety of conditions. They found that the internalization of one's worth being defined by one's attractiveness "plays an important role in the development of mental health issues in young women," including disordered eating (p. 66). And that makes sense to me: If you believe that your worth is tied up in how beautiful you are (and if beauty is related to a white, able, cisheteronormative standard of thinness in your social context), *of course* you might fall prey to eating disorders!

Simply put, when our bodies are being surveilled, socially or interpersonally, we learn to surveil ourselves. This is especially true the more marginalized we are: Fat women, trans women, disabled women, women of color, and more are under increased social (and therefore, individual) surveillance. The male gaze, white gaze, and so on – the perspectives of beauty that are governed by people and institutions in dominance – are powerful judgments rooted in systemic oppression. And when we internalize that way of seeing other people and turn it on ourselves, the results can be disastrous.

SEXUAL HARASSMENT

When I think about sexual harassment, I often think about catcalling – and I remember vividly the first time that I was catcalled.

I was ten or eleven, waiting on my stoop for my dad, who was dragging me along on an errand with him. It was springtime, but I was chomping on a candy cane leftover from Christmas, sliding it against my tongue and feeling my head filled with the all-encompassing sensation of peppermint. A man walked by and he casually said to me, "I wish you would suck me like that." I remember how coolly he said it – tossed it to me – as if it were as perfectly natural as "hello." At the time, I had no idea what he meant; but just the same, it made me feel filthy – embarrassed and regretful.

This experience was, of course, horrendous. And although I'd like to believe that I was much too young to incur such a response, unfortunately, most women I've talked to about their first experiences with catcalling name puberty as the start of it, too.

Women are indoctrinated into objectification – and accepting it as a way of life – before we've even had a chance to explore our own authentic, autonomous sexuality. Of course that has an effect on our relationships to our bodies.

As such, objectification has been supported as a possible influence in eating disorder development (Calogero & Thompson, 2009; Slater & Tiggemann, 2010). For example, one 2002 study concluded that women's experiences of sexual harassment could predict eating disorder symptoms, so long as sexual assault was included in the data (Harned & Fitzgerald, 2002). Further, a 2013 study found that body-based harassment, defined as objectifying comments toward a girl's body, had a negative effect on 12- to 14-year-old girls' eating patterns and could contribute to eating disorder development (Holman, Johnson, & Lucier, 2013).

Specifically, another 2013 study suggested that this relationship might be mediated by self-surveillance in regard to how one looks (Petersen & Hyde, 2013): Girls who experienced sexual harassment were more likely to engage in self-surveillance, which resulted in more disordered eating patterns.

When girls are made to feel more self-conscious about their bodies, especially at various other intersections of marginalized identity, they may be more likely to engage in disordered eating to mitigate that discomfort.

SEXUAL ASSAULT AND ABUSE

Before we can dig into a conversation about sexual assault and abuse, it's important to make sure we're on the same page in terms of definitions of these violations.

Of course, the legal definitions differ state by state and country by country – and as such, if you're interested in how these terms are defined by the law where you are, I suggest looking it up.

Here, I want to tell you how I'm using these words, based on my experiences with research in Human Sexuality Studies and employment in sexual assault and domestic violence prevention and intervention services:

- *Sexual assault* is any act of physical touch that is unwanted. Touching someone in a sexual manner without their explicit, authentic consent is sexual assault.
- *Rape* is a type of sexual assault that is defined by unwanted penetration of any object in any orifice, especially in the vagina or anus, or oral penetration with a sexual organ.
- *Sexual abuse* is the repeated, patterned, manipulative use of (often unwanted) sexual behavior to gain power and control over another person.

- *Childhood sexual abuse* is the experience of sexual abuse enacted by an adult on a minor.
- *Incest* is defined as a sexual contact between family members. While incest is not inherently assaultive or abusive, it is a common form of abuse, especially among children.

Please note that these are basic, foundational definitions. I encourage you to learn more about these acts from a reputable source, such as your local advocacy organization or RAINN.

Many women with eating disorders have had experiences with sexual trauma in their pasts (Kong & Bernstein, 2009; Tagay, Schlottbohm, Reyes-Rodriguez, Repic, & Senf, 2014). For example, rape survivors may be more likely than others to meet eating disorder diagnostic criteria: One 2004 study found that 53% of their 40 female sexual trauma survivors experienced eating disorders, as compared to just 6% of 32 women with no sexual trauma history (Faravelli, Giugni, Salvatori, & Ricca, 2004).

One reason for this may be the mediating factor of post-traumatic stress disorder (PTSD) (Dubosc et al., 2012). That is, it may not be the sexual assault in and of itself that may affect women's eating habits, but, rather, the resulting capital-T trauma. In a survey of 296 French women, researchers found that "PTSD symptoms fully mediated the effect of early adult sexual assault on disordered eating" (Dubosc et al., 2012, p. 5). Similarly, another 2012 study found a relationship between sexual trauma, PTSD, and eating disorders in female military veterans (Forman-Hoffman, Mengeling, Booth, Torner, & Sadler, 2012).

Further, childhood sexual abuse (CSA) specifically has been explored as a potential connection (Dyer et al., 2013; Steiger et al., 2010). A 2001 study found that women with a history of CSA were much more likely to meet diagnostic criteria for an eating disorder, especially if they had also experienced sexual violence in adulthood (Wonderlich et al., 2001). This research also showed that in 92% of the cases where women experienced both CSA and eating disorder symptoms, the abuse preceded the eating disorder.

Indeed, in relation to eating disorders and sexual functioning, CSA could be a mediating factor. A 2013 study reported that those with eating disorders who also report a history of CSA exhibit "profound uneasiness" in body perception and sexual functioning (Castellini et al., 2013, p. 2190). More specifically, a 1995 study pointed out that incest survivors have a higher rate of eating disorders (47%) than otherwise sexually abused clients (22%), unaffected incest survivors (24%), and those who had never been abused (17%) (Mallinckrodt, McCreary, & Robertson, 1995).

It's important to note that despite the popular myth that CSA and eating disorders are causationally related, results in the vein of CSA and eating disorders have often been inconclusive (Smolak & Murnen, 2002). Eating disorders absolutely can be triggered by trauma – and sexual violence, including CSA, absolutely can be traumatic – but we cannot assume a clear, causal relationship.

AUTONOMY AND CONSENT

In conversations with participants in my study, this topic came up a lot. In fact, one of the findings of my study was that trust and autonomy were the biggest factors in whether someone interpreted touch from a subject standpoint (as an active participant) or an object standpoint (as a passive participant).

That is, when my participants were engaging with people with whom they had a trusting relationship, who respected their boundaries, and who adjusted their expectations accordingly, they felt that they had more control over who touched them and how. When that choice was explicitly present – when they felt open to accepting, rejecting, or initiating touch on their own terms – they were more likely to express touch as positive. But when others made assumptions about their comfort levels – like standing too close to them or hugging them without permission – they felt violated and associated those interactions with fear and anxiety. This was true whether we were talking about sexual contact or sensual contact. The line between pleasure and violation was in the level of control they had over the situation.

Adra had a brilliant, dichotomous way of explaining this experience: "I like touching other people. I just don't like other people to touch me."

Consent – and comfort declining – made the biggest difference. When participants felt that they had control over their experiences, they were far more likely to experience the touch as positive. "As long as I'm comfortable with them, and feel safe with them, and don't feel like they're going to judge me, or as long as I like them and want to be touched by them, [it's fine]. It has to be someone that I know and love," Kaylee said.

Perhaps touch – whether sexual or sensual – in and of itself, is not the issue to be concerned with, but rather how that touch shows up in our lives. For my participants, within a trusting relationship wherein their boundaries are respected and emotional intimacy is explored, they expressed an ability to engage in and enjoy touch. And that can be a powerful reclamation from the common narrative that women with anorexia *just don't enjoy sex.*

It makes sense that eating disorders, often understood as extreme reclamation of control over one's body, especially as maladaptive coping mechanisms to deal with trauma, can be connected to sexual violence.

Furthermore, it makes sense that a group of people for whom obsessive control is often a common personality trait would express a deep, unwavering need for consent.

Our experiences in our bodies are interconnected. And this is what makes a complex understanding of sexuality so vital – not so that we can treat people, least of all ourselves, as problems to be solved, but so that we can respect and honor those complexities and the relationships that they form.

REFERENCES

Calogero, R. M., & Thompson, J. K. (2009). Sexual self-esteem in American and British college women: Relations with self-objectification and eating problems. *Sex Roles, 60*(3/4), 160–173.

Castellini, G., Lo Sauro, C., Lelli, L., Godini, L., Vignozzi, L., Rellini, A. H., … Ricca, V. (2013). Childhood sexual abuse moderates the relationship between sexual functioning and eating disorder psychopathology in anorexia nervosa and bulimia nervosa: A 1-year follow-up study. *Journal of Sexual Medicine, 10*(9), 2190–2200.

Dubosc, A., Capitaine, M., Franko, D. L., Bui, R., Brunet, A., Chabrol, H., … Rodgers, R. F. (2012). Early adult sexual assault and disordered eating: The mediating role of posttraumatic stress symptoms. *Journal of Traumatic Stress, 25*(1), 50–56.

Dyer, A., Borgmann, E., Feldman, R. E., Jr., Kleindienst, N., Prieve, K. Bohus, M., & Vocks, S. (2013). Body image disturbance in patients with borderline personality disorder: Impact of eating disorders and perceived childhood sexual abuse. *Body Image, 10*(2), 220–225.

Faravelli, C., Giugni, A., Salvatori, S., & Ricca, V. (2004). Psychopathology after rape. *American Journal of Psychiatry, 161*(8), 1483–1485. Retrieved from http://www.ncbi.nlm.nih.gov/pubmed/15285977

Forman-Hoffman, V. L., Mengeling, M., Booth, B. M., Torner, J., & Sadler, A. G. (2012). Eating disorders, post-traumatic stress, and sexual trauma in women veterans. *Military Medicine, 177*(10), 1161–1168.

Fredrickson, B. L., & Roberts, T. (1997). Objectification theory: Toward understanding women's lived experiences and mental health risks. *Psychology of Women Quarterly, 21*(2), 173–206.

Harned, M. S., & Fitzgerald, L. F. (2002). Understanding a link between sexual harassment and eating disorder symptoms: A mediational analysis. *Journal of Consulting and Clinical Psychology, 70*(5), 1170–1181.

Holman, M. J., Johnson, J., & Lucier, M. (2013). Sticks and stones: The multifarious effects of body-based harassment on young girls' healthy lifestyle choices. *Sport, Education, and Society, 18*(4), 527–549.

Kong, S., & Bernstein, K. (2009). Childhood trauma as a predictor of eating psychopathology and its mediating variables in patients with eating disorders. *Journal of Clinical Nursing, 18*(13), 1897–1907.

Mallinckrodt, B., McCreary, B. A., & Robertson, A. K. (1995). Co-occurrence of eating disorders and incest: The role of attachment, family environment, and social competencies. *Journal of Counseling Psychology, 42*(2), 178–186.

Moradi, B., Dirks, D., & Matteson, A. V. (2005). Roles of sexual objectification experiences and internalization of standards of beauty in eating disorder symptomatology: A test and extension of objectification theory. *Journal of Counseling Psychology, 52*(3), 420–428.

Petersen, J. L., & Hyde, J. S. (2013). Peer sexual harassment and disordered eating in early adolescence. *Developmental Psychology, 49*(1), 184–195.

Slater, A., & Tiggemann, M. (2010). Body image and disordered eating in adolescent girls and boys: A test of objectification theory. *Sex Roles, 63*(1), 42–49.

Smolak, L., & Murnen, S. K. (2002). A meta-analytic examination of the relationship between child sexual abuse and eating disorders. *International Journal of Eating Disorders, 31*(2), 136–150.

Steiger, H., Richardson, J., Schmitz, N., Israel, M., Bruce, K. R., & Gauvin, L. (2010). Trait-defined eating-disorder subtypes and history of childhood abuse. *International Journal of Eating Disorders, 43*(5), 428–432.

Szymanski, D. M., Moffitt, L. B., & Carr, E. R. (2011). Sexual objectification of women: Advances to theory and research. *The Counseling Psychologist, 39*(1), 6–38.

Tagay, S., Schlottbohm, E., Reyes-Rodriguez, M. L., Repic, N., & Senf, W. (2014). Eating disorders, trauma, PTSD, and psychosocial resources. *Eating Disorders, 22*(1), 33–49.

Tiggemann, M., & Williams, E. (2012). The role of self-objectification in disordered eating, depressed mood, and sexual functioning among women: A comprehensive test of objectification theory. *Psychology of Women Quarterly, 36*(1), 66–75.

Wonderlich, S. A., Crosby, R. D., Mitchell, J. E., Thompson, K. M., Redlin, J., Demuth, G.,…Haseltine, B. (2001). Eating disturbance and sexual trauma in childhood and adulthood. *International Journal of Eating Disorders, 30*(4), 401–412.

Identity

Chapter 6

My brother once told me that, in a pinch, when someone asked him what I studied, he said that I studied gender and LGBTQIA+ issues. He wasn't terribly off – but he wasn't on the nose, either.

It wasn't an unsurprising flub to me, though, because many people hear the word *sexuality* and conflate it with *orientation*, just one aspect of identity.

What's funny about identity is that there is a prevailing assumption that it's only those of us who are marginalized who hold them. Folks don't think of *man* or *white* or *straight* as identities, even though they are – and important, powerful ones at that. Those identities play a huge role in how those who hold them move through the world, including sexually.

People scoff at quote-unquote "identity politics," but acknowledging that our identities affect our worldviews and experiences, including in sexuality, isn't actually offensive – or even interesting, to tell the truth. If you ask me, we need to add a sixth circle to this model: "Social Location," which addresses how our overlapping experiences of both power and oppression affect our experiences of sexuality. But that's another book, I guess.

Within the realm of sexuality, when we talk about identity, we're talking about *sexual* identity specifically: experiences of orientation, gender identity, and gender roles.

According to Advocates for Youth (2018, para. 14), sexual identity is "a person's understanding of who [they are] sexually" – which includes their experience of sexual orientation (which is determined by which gender[s] a person is primarily attracted to, if any), gender identity (one's innate sense of gender, or lack thereof), and the gender roles that they perform (socially constructed behaviors that are assigned gender).

Here, I'm going to focus on marginalized identities (queer women, transgender women, and femininity) not because privileged identities don't influence sexuality, but because I would rather center the marginalized – and compare privileged experiences to them. Too often, we do the opposite, centering the privileged and assuming that experience to be the standard.

This is especially important because LGBTQIA+ people have not, historically, been included in general eating disorder research.

Much of the research that *has* explored this population in regard to eating disorders has focused on the experiences of gay, bisexual, and queer men, concluding that this group is more likely than their straight counterparts to experience negative body image and develop eating disorders (Austin et al., 2004; Strong, Williamson, Netemeyer, & Geer, 2000). Much less has been explored in regard to queer and trans women. Worse, almost no research exists that addresses how non-binary, intersex, and asexual people experience eating disorders – something that must be remedied. However, eating disorders may disproportionately affect some parts of the LGBTQIA+ population because of the distinct pressures with which we're faced.

According to the National Eating Disorders Association (2015), some of the unique stress factors that LGBTQIA+ people face include coming out, fear of familial rejection, internalized queer- and transantagonism, bullying, and other violence. These additional oppressive stress factors may impact the likelihood of developing anxiety, depression, low self-esteem, and harmful coping mechanisms, such as substance abuse, all of which frequently co-occur with and contribute to eating disorders.

These risk factors are combined with a lack of support systems and culturally competent treatment: People who are trained to support LGBTQIA+ people are not well-versed in eating disorders, and people who are trained to assist in eating disorders aren't prepared for the special considerations needed for LGBTQIA+ populations (Waldron, Semerjian, & Kauer, 2009).

The combination of these factors can be dangerous in the resulting inability for LGBTQIA+ people to receive treatment. So it's important that we take time within eating disorder conversations to focus on these populations.

LESBIAN, BISEXUAL, AND QUEER WOMEN

Here is what we know: First and foremost – and as a bisexual woman myself, I think it's really important to point it out – there is no significant difference in eating disorder prevalence between straight and queer women (Ray, 2006).

Yes, early research suggested that eating disorders occur in 5–10% of straight women and 2–3% of lesbian women (Costin, 1999; Settles, Hanks, & Sussman, 1993). But more recent research says that straight and queer women are equally likely to develop eating disorders (Feldman & Meyer, 2007).

When parsing out specific eating disorders, some research shows that lesbian women are less likely than their straight counterparts to develop anorexia nervosa, but are more likely to develop bulimia nervosa and binge eating disorder (Millner, 2004; Wichstrøm, 2006). Similarly, binge eating and purging have been found to be more common in lesbian, bisexual, and "mostly heterosexual" women than in their straight-identified peers (Austin et al., 2004).

Despite this research, though, many people perceive queer women's orientations as protection against eating disorder development (Swain, 2006). You heard me: There is a prevailing assumption that *by virtue of being queer,* some women may be unlikely to experience eating disorders.

Uh, what?

Here's the deal: It's sometimes believed that because lesbian women, in particular, but also queer women as a whole, belong to a sociocultural community outside of, and perhaps even counter to, the dominant culture, we're less likely to internalize the feminine ideals presented by that dominant group and more likely to redefine ideals on our own terms.

That is, the belief is that because queer women form identity and community counter to the male gaze, that we somehow escape it entirely.

It's been shown, for instance, that lesbian culture, as compared to the dominant culture, lacks the same emphasis on physical appearance in regard to mate selection, which some propose may affect the rates of body dissatisfaction and disordered eating in this population (Morrison, Morrison, & Sager, 2004; Strong et al., 2000).

A 2004 study by Austin et al. found that their lesbian and bisexual participants were more satisfied with their bodies and less concerned with the media's portrayal of women's attractiveness. More specifically, a 1999 study by Ludwig and Brownell found that lesbian and bisexual women who identify as feminine have significantly worse body image than those who identify as masculine or androgynous.

This may point to gender presentation as a significant factor in the likelihood of eating disorder development in lesbian, bisexual, and queer women; however, as will be explored further in the "Femininity" section, the long-standing myth that femininity is a risk factor in eating disorder development may be grossly overstated.

This all makes sense. However, it very clearly ignores the intersection of gender in this conversation.

In 2011, Jones and Malson explored how lesbian and bisexual women make meaning of their eating disorder experiences, and interesting conclusions came from their interviews: overall, participants attributed *both* similar *and* different meaning to their experiences of anorexia and bulimia nervosas as their straight counterparts. While "a search for identity, an exertion of self-control, and a pursuit of feminine beauty" played roles in their experiences, they also expressed the significance of their eating disorders developing as a "response to the stress and uncertainty of not fulfilling heteronormative expectations and/or as a way of avoiding their sexuality by focusing instead on food or by 'looking straight'" (p. 18).

Indeed, their intersections of gender and orientation mattered to them: They experience life as women in society, and are therefore susceptible to what that means overall, but they also specifically experience life as lesbian, bisexual, and queer women in society, which complicates their experience of womanhood and adds distinct pressures.

In my research, most of my participants were LGBTQIA+: Only three of my 20 interviewees identified as straight. Participants' queerness (or sexual identity overall) rarely came up in conversation. When it did, though, the feelings expressed were strong.

For example, some participants, particularly those who have had sexual experiences with multiple genders, expressed a stronger distrust for men: "I feel like it's different with women," Inari said. One participant even discussed her experience being married to a man, while feeling that she's a lesbian, and the complexity this adds to her life.

Multiple participants also wanted to discuss asexuality. While some pointed out that despite their lack of desire, they don't necessarily identify as asexual, others wore the label proudly. Three participants identified as asexual in the initial survey; others toyed with the idea in their interviews. For example, Lin explained, "I think that when I was in the restrictive mindset, it was like my sexuality shut down completely…I just became sort of asexual at that point."

While orientation wasn't a beacon for exploration in my own interviews, it still came up for people as connected to their sexual experiences. Especially for those who are marginalized, orientation can be a blatant and obvious connection to their eating disorders.

TRANSGENDER WOMEN

In 2015, Diemer, Grant, Munn-Chernoff, Patterson, and Duncan conducted a study believed to include "the largest number of transgender participants ever to be surveyed" about eating disorders – with a sample size of 289,024 college students of various sexual orientations and gender identities (p. 147).

Yeah.

Wow.

Overall, they found that transgender youth are at an increased risk for eating disorder development, as transgender students were most likely to have been diagnosed with an eating disorder in the past year – yes, even compared to straight, cisgender women. More specifically, transgender participants were more likely to have engaged in compensatory behaviors, such as the use of diet pills, self-induced vomiting, and laxative abuse.

Importantly, though, there are various potential explanations for this relationship.

For example, transgender people are more likely to have contact with mental health professionals who could diagnose them with eating disorders. A 2001 study by Grant et al. showed that 75% of transgender people receive counseling already. Further, this population experiences higher rates of various mental health issues, including attempted suicide, which also makes them more likely to be seeking psychological support (Clements-Nolle, Marx, & Katz, 2006). This is not, of course, to suggest that the experience of being transgender is, in and of itself, a mental health issue. It is unequivocally not. However, because transgender people are often made to receive signatures from mental health professionals to move forward with various biological transitions, and because of the trauma associated with oppression, many transgender people may already be connected to mental health professionals. And those professionals are the exact people from whom many folks receive eating disorder diagnoses in the first place.

Minority stress, or the experience of oppression, may also make transgender people more likely to resort to disordered eating, especially as it relates to cisnormative beauty ideals (Ålgars, Santtila, & Sandnabba, 2010; Vocks, Stahn, Loenser, & Legenbauer, 2009).

According to Diemer et al. (2015, p. 147), "transgender individuals may use disordered eating behaviors to suppress or accentuate particularly gendered features." And transgender women in particular may use weight loss as a way to conform to feminine beauty ideals (Ålgars et al., 2010). Indeed, a 2012 study by Ålgars, Alanko, Santtila, and Sandnabba found that a majority (70%) of their transgender participants experienced disordered eating, and they found that this was especially in regard to "striving 'for thinness as an attempt to suppress features' or to 'accentuate features' in accordance with their gender identity."

For transgender women, and transgender women of color in particular, conforming to cisnormative beauty standards may also be a means of survival – hate crimes, including murder, committed against this group are horrifyingly prevalent – and "passing" to outsiders as their gender without question or suspicion may create a sense of safety.

However, the psychological experience of body dysphoria, or the stress or discomfort in one's body due to its misalignment with one's gender identity, may play a large role in body dissatisfaction among transgender women who experience that phenomenon. One 2009 study by Khoosal, Langham, Palmer, Terry, and Minajagi found that for transgender women who desired it, gender affirmation surgical procedures decreased their levels of body dissatisfaction. This echoes a 2004 study by Winston, Archaya, Chaudhuri, and Fellowes that found similar results. Further, after gender affirmation surgery, many transgender women report feelings of improved attractiveness, lower insecurity, and fewer body image concerns (Kraemer, Delsignore, Schnyder, & Hepp, 2008).

Despite these associations, though, as well as the need for more resources for marginalized populations, transgender women are rarely explicitly included in general studies on eating disorders.

This must change in order to find people the support they need, but it also must change in order to fully represent womanhood and the complexities therein.

Even in my own study, where two women identified as transgender, three as non-binary, and two as intersex, this conversation wasn't had explicitly. Of course, like with other topics of identity that weren't addressed directly, this is mostly because we were talking about touch specifically, and participants may have felt that it wasn't an appropriate forum for discussing their experiences with gender.

But in 2014, Drummond and Brotman wrote that the importance of addressing various oppressions "at individual and institutional levels" in order to "address the intersectional nature of identity and the impacts of occupying multiple marginalized positions" is necessary in working with all marginalized populations – and this includes queer and trans women (p. 533).

FEMININITY

It has long been assumed that the more closely women, or people in general, associate with femininity, the more likely they are to develop anorexia nervosa. Partly, this is due to the development of understanding anorexia nervosa as an illness: From the beginning, it had always been addressed only in women, and a very particular, privileged subset of women, at that.

However, a 2011 study by Till explored how gender has been quantified in regard to investigating anorexia nervosa, and it's worth a look: In this research, it's noted that the continued assumptions about the association between anorexia nervosa and femininity may possibly be linked to long-standing researcher bias more than anything else.

Till (2011) reviewed how the introduction of gender identity scales seemed to prove objectively that femininity is a risk factor for eating disorder development, but points out that this could have been subjective on the part of the researcher: "Gender identity scales gave psychiatrists a way of transforming the complex, dynamic, processual phenomenon of gender into a static, individualized, quantifiable one" (p. 440). This should bring about some concerns.

In fact, the work of Bem (1974) and Constantinople (1973) found that these scales were somewhat subjective: They often associated traditionally "masculine" traits with well-being by only including socially desirable masculine traits (think: *strength* or *leadership*). Instead, these scales need to allow for both masculine and feminine traits to exist in all genders, rather than associating masculinity with men and femininity with women – and showing preference for the former.

Till (2011) noted that when scales that allow for more fluidity in gender roles have been applied to anorexia nervosa, "such nuances [are not] evident" (p. 441).

Indeed, more current research exploring gender roles and eating disorders have varying results. A 2001 study by Meyer, Blisset, and Oldfield found that femininity was a risk factor for, and masculinity a protective factor in, eating disorder development; a 2005 study by Hepp, Spindler, and Milos also found a correlation between higher levels of masculinity and lower levels of eating disorder symptoms (but, notably, didn't find that higher levels of femininity led to eating disorder symptomology). But Januszek (2007) found *no* significant difference between women with anorexia nervosa and unaffected women in terms of idealized beliefs about gender roles (although the group of women with anorexia nervosa did have significantly more feminine traits than the unaffected group).

As such, gender roles may or may not play a significant role in the development of eating disorders – the jury, as they say, is still out. And we would do well not to make assumptions either way.

What this survey of identity *can* tell us, though, is that eating disorders are complicated, and how we've perceived them in the scientific community has shifted significantly over time.

The more we can dedicate ourselves to exploring these ideas, the better the research will be. One way that we can do that is by making sure that we code for identity in our work, and that we do so with nuance.

REFERENCES

Advocates for Youth. (2018). An explanation of the Circles of Sexuality. Retrieved from http://www.advocatesforyouth.org/for-professionals/lesson-plans professionals/200

Ålgars, M., Alanko, K., Santtila, P., & Sandnabba, N. K. (2012). Disordered eating and gender identity disorder: A qualitative study. *Eating Disorders, 20*(4), 300–311.

Ålgars, M., Santtila, P., & Sandnabba, N. K. (2010). Conflicted gender identity, body dissatisfaction, and disordered eating in adult men and women. *Sex Roles, 63*(1), 118–125.

Austin, S. B., Ziyadeh, N., Kahn, J. A., Camargo, C. A., Jr., Colditz, G. A., & Field, A. E. (2004). Sexual orientation, weight concerns, and eating-disordered behaviors in adolescent girls and boys. *Psychiatry, 43*(9), 1115–1123.

Bem, S. L. (1974). The measurement of psychological androgyny. *Journal of Consulting and Clinical Psychology, 42*(2), 155–162.

Clements-Nolle, K., Marx, R., & Katz, M. (2006). Attempted suicide among transgender persons: The influence of gender-based discrimination and victimization. *Journal of Homosexuality, 51*(3), 53–69.

Constantinople, A. (1973). Masculinity-femininity: An exception to a famous dictum? *Psychological Bulletin, 80*(5), 389–407.

Costin, C. (1999). *The eating disorder sourcebook: A comprehensive guide to the causes, treatments, and prevention of eating disorders.* New York, NY: McGraw-Hill Professional.

Diemer, E. W., Grant, J. D., Munn-Chernoff, M. A., Patterson, D. A., & Duncan, A. E. (2015). Gender identity, sexual orientation, and eating-related pathology in a national sample of college students. *Journal of Adolescent Health, 57*(2), 144–149.

Drummond, J. D., & Brotman, S. (2014). Intersecting and embodied identities: A queer woman's experience of disability and sexuality. *Sexuality and Disability, 32*(4), 533–549.

Feldman, M. B., & Meyer, I. H. (2007). Eating disorders in diverse lesbian, gay, and bisexual populations. *International Journal of Eating Disorders, 40*(3), 218–226.

Grant, J. M., Mottet, L. A., Tanis, J., Harrison, J., Herman, J. L., & Keisling, M. (2001). *Injustice at every turn: A report of the national transgender discrimination survey.* Washington, DC: National Center for Transgender Equality and National Gay and Lesbian Task Force.

Hepp, U., Spindler, A., & Milos, G. (2005). Eating disorder symptomology and gender role orientation. *International Journal of Eating Disorders, 37*(3), 227–233.

Januszek, K. (2007). Some aspects of sexual identity of girls suffering from anorexia nervosa. *Archives of Psychiatry and Psychotherapy, 9*(3), 53–62.

Jones, R., & Malson, H. (2011). A critical exploration of lesbian perspectives on eating disorders. *Psychology and Sexuality, 4*(1), 1–27.

Khoosal, D., Langham, C., Palmer, B., Terry, T., & Minajagi, M. (2009). Features of eating disorder among male-to-female transsexuals. *Sexual and Relationship Therapy, 24*(2), 217–229.

Kraemer, B., Delsignore, A., Schnyder, U., & Hepp, U. (2008). Body image and transexualism. *Psychopathology, 41*(2), 96–100.

Ludwig, M. R., & Brownell, K. D. (1999). Lesbians, bisexual women, and body image: An investigation of gender roles and social group affiliation. *International Journal of Eating Disorders, 25*(1), 89–97.

Meyer, C., Blisset, J., & Oldfield, C. (2001). Sexual orientation and eating psychopathology: The role of masculinity and femininity. *International Journal of Eating Disorders, 29*(3), 314–318.

Millner, R. E. (2004). The experience of lesbians who have a history of binge eating disorder: A qualitative investigation. *Dissertation Abstracts International: Section B: The Sciences and Engineering, 65*(3-B).

Morrison, M. A., Morrison, T. G., & Sager, C. L. (2004). Does body dissatisfaction differ between gay men and lesbian women and heterosexual men and women? A meta- analytic review. *Body Image, 1*(2), 127–138.

National Eating Disorders Association. (2015). *Eating disorders in LGBT populations.* Retrieved from http://www.nationaleatingdisorders.org/eating-disorders-lgbt-populations

Ray, N. (2006). *Lesbian, gay, bisexual, and transgender youth: An epidemic of homelessness.* National Gay and Lesbian Taskforce. Retrieved from http://www.thetaskforce.org/static_html/downloads/HomelessYouth.pdf

Settles, B. H., Hanks, R. S., & Sussman, M. B. (1993). *American families and the future: analyses of possible destinies.* New York, NY: Routledge.

Strong, S. M., Williamson, D. A., Netemeyer, R. G., & Geer, J. H. (2000). Eating disorder symptoms and concerns about body differ as a function of gender and sexual orientation. *Journal of Social and Clinical Psychology, 19*(2), 240–256.

Swain, P. (2006). *New developments in eating disorder research.* New York, NY: Nova Science.

Till, C. (2011). The quantification of gender: Anorexia nervosa and femininity. *Health Sociology Review, 20*(4), 437–449.

Vocks, S., Stahn, C., Loenser, K., & Legenbauer, T. (2009). Eating and body image disturbances in male-to-female and female-to-male transsexuals. *Archives of Sexual Behavior, 38*(3), 364–377.

Waldron, J. J., Semerjian, T., & Kauer, K. (2009). Doing "drag": Applying queer-feminist theory to the body image and eating disorders across sexual orientation and gender identity. In J. J. Reel & K. A. Beals (Eds.), *The hidden faces of eating disorders and body image* (pp. 63–81). Reston, VA: American Alliance for Health Physical.

Wichstrøm, L. (2006). Sexual orientation as a risk factor for bulimic symptoms. *International Journal of Eating Disorders, 39*(6), 448–453.

Winston, A. P., Archaya, S., Chaudhuri, S., & Fellowes, L. (2004). Anorexia nervosa and gender identity disorder in biologic males: A report of two cases. *International Journal of Eating Disorders, 36*(1), 109–113.

Intimacy

Chapter 7

When I give presentations on intimate partner violence (IPV) at universities, I often start the conversation at the word *intimate*. Partly, this is a way to suss out IPV from its umbrella term, domestic violence (DV), since many people conflate the two. "When you hear the word *intimate*," I ask the students in the room, as I pace across my (often makeshift) stage, "what do you think of?"

And they always give me the answer that I'm looking for: sex. This allows for a great jumping off point for exploring how violence against sexual and romantic partners is a specific type of DV, with its own set of dynamics.

But from there, I always have to take a step back to help my audience excavate more meanings for the word *intimate* and, in doing so, discovering more ways in which IPV can show up.

Because intimacy is *not* inherently sexual.

Intimacy is about *closeness*.

According to Advocates for Youth (2018, para. 8), intimacy is "the ability to be emotionally close to another human being and to accept closeness in return." Intimacy is less about sexual connection and more about the emotional aspect of relating to another person. This includes sharing, caring, liking and loving, emotional risk-taking, and vulnerability.

The experience of close relationships with others plays a large role in our daily lives – and is central to the human experience. Even Aristotle (350 BCE), who believed happiness to be the ultimate purpose of human existence, contemplated the necessity of intimacy, suggesting that human beings are social by nature. Aristotle believed that people form relationships based on three factors: utility (the assistance that other people provide), virtue (attraction to others' moral character), and pleasure (a sense of joy when with others) – and that all of these types of relationships play a part in satisfying the human need for social interaction.

Much later, Maslow (1943, 1954) introduced his hierarchy of needs, an idea that was stolen from Blackfoot Nation people and Westernized to put self-actualization at the top, rather than at the bottom (Blackstock, 2011). Due to white supremacy and colonization in academia, Maslow's version remains the foundational model for understanding our biological, psychological, and social needs. However, both models explore how close relationships with others are a basic need of human existence. Maslow argued that people need to feel a sense of belonging, acceptance, and love in their social groups; otherwise, people will be susceptible to feelings of loneliness, which can be psychologically damaging. Blackfoot Nation names community actualization – or collective fulfillment – as an endeavor toward the ultimate goal of cultural perpetuity (Blackstock, 2011). Close, strong relationships with others, though contextualized differently, are arguably universally valued.

Intimacy – which includes everything from sharing secrets and giggles over crushes at middle school sleepovers to sitting down with a new partner to explain past trauma – is a foundational aspect of human interaction, including for women with anorexia nervosa.

EMOTIONAL CLOSENESS

Unfortunately, little research has attempted to explore the ways in which women with anorexia nervosa experience intimacy in their relationships, particularly from a qualitative standpoint.

Some literature has pointed to an overall observation that women with eating disorders show a higher likelihood of negative relational experiences and a decreased likelihood of engaging in romantic or sexual relationships at all (Ghizzani & Montomoli, 2000). However, they've also been clear to point out the difficulty in pinpointing specific trends, due to an underdevelopment of research in this area.

However, in the early 2000s, two important studies by Newton, Boblin, Brown, and Ciliska (2005, 2006) explored the ways in which women with anorexia nervosa make meaning out of their experiences with intimacy within romantic relationships, providing what is currently the most in-depth source of information on the topic, despite a small sample size.

These two phenomenological studies surveyed 11 straight women, aged 19–42, with anorexia nervosa through in-depth, semi-structured interviews. And two important themes emerged: first, the opposing themes of engagement and distancing, which drove both the changes in and the maintenance of the participants' romantic relationships; then, themes of emotional closeness (including disclosure, trust and acceptance, and feeling known), physical closeness (including both sexual and non-sexual expressions), and companionship (including recreational activity and parenting).

With little past research to guide their study, the authors found that participants were able "to identify what intimacy meant to them, their experiences with intimacy, and what they needed within their romantic relationships to be intimate" (Newton et al., 2006, p. 43), reflective of prior research on intimacy in unaffected populations (Buhrmester & Furman, 1987; Jourard, 1971).

However, while in many ways, this sample of women with anorexia nervosa mirrored the experiences of the general population, it's important to note that "the women's intimate experiences were often mediated by their eating disorders" (Newton et al., 2006, p. 49).

In 2006, Newton et al. found, overall, that the "intimate experiences of the participants were diverse," but that many of them desired more intimacy than they were experiencing in their relationships (p. 46). This may be tied to the expression of more need for touch nurturance in women with anorexia nervosa, which will be discussed in detail in the next chapter.

One significant theme that emerged from these interviews was that, for women with anorexia nervosa, disclosure plays a large role in the ability to feel close to a partner – including disclosure of the eating disorder itself.

The participants explained that in order to build trust in their relationships, they needed to feel free to discuss their experiences with anorexia nervosa with their partners. More specifically, some women expressed that it was important to them that their partners were "interested in listening to and trying to better understand their experience" (p. 47), and others named that their partners could never fully grasp the experience of an eating disorder without having experienced it. Regardless, most of the participants felt that congruent disclosure (that is, both partners feeling comfortable sharing with one another) led to more emotional closeness.

This emotional closeness was how participants defined "engagement" with their partners, while physical connectedness (in this context, sex) was deprioritized. In order to initiate a relationship successfully, the participants sought connection and attention as a "reinforcing factor to maintain a perceived female ideal" (Newton et al., 2005, p. 321). For a relationship to transition into a safe space for disclosure, especially of the eating disorder, participants felt that trust and support were necessary. Only at this point could more open dialogue occur. The women felt that this was important so that they could express their needs, especially in relation to their eating disorder; however, some women, particularly those whose eating disorder symptoms were severe, were less likely to disclose, out of fear that it would add stress to the relationship.

A common refrain that came up in interviews with my own participants was that of eating disorder-induced isolation: Many participants talked about how they isolated themselves from those around them during their eating disorder, partly because they didn't want relationships to interrupt their disorders, and partly because of guilt and shame.

"Any kind of close relationships just got so fucking complex," Winnie said of her experience with an eating disorder. Talia detailed, "It can be really hard for me to feel like I can trust other people...like I can connect. I still feel a fair amount of shame about the eating disorder itself and have a hard time talking about it with friends."

All of which brings up the question of whether women with anorexia nervosa tend to display personality traits that lead them *both* to their eating disorder *and* to avoiding intimacy, or if the eating disorder itself affects the level of intimacy in their relationships.

A 2013 study by Brockmeyer et al. examined whether autonomy disturbances (that is, struggles with normative motivation for independence) exist in women with anorexia nervosa, and found that this population had a higher motivation for avoiding dependency, as well as less endeavoring for intimacy, than unaffected women. That is, the common autonomy disturbance for this population isn't that they have too *little* motivation for independence, but perhaps too *much*.

In this study, women in recovery were more motivated toward intimacy and more satisfied in their intimate relationships than women who were currently struggling with an eating disorder. This suggests that while "a pronounced motive of avoiding dependency may be a vulnerability factor for anorexia nervosa that is disorder-specific and trait-like" (p. 278), it may be more connected to the presentation of the eating disorder, rather than the people who exhibit them.

This means, perhaps, that less endeavoring for intimate relationships may not be "a stable characteristic of women with a history" of anorexia nervosa, but rather, is connected to the disorder itself (p. 285).

ATTACHMENT THEORY

A brief exploration of attachment theory (Bowlby, 1969) can be helpful in situating the relationship between women with anorexia nervosa and intimacy, particularly because insecure attachment is such a common experience for people with eating disorders.

Attachment theory is, essentially, a model through which personality development can be understood. Specifically, it aims to elucidate the ways in which one's experience in infancy, in relation to the start of social and psychological conditioning from a primary caregiver, creates a foundation for one's long-term interpersonal relationships.

Beginning with the level of a baby's development of trust that it will be cared for, attachment grows to explain how people respond to interpersonal hurt, separation, and threat (Waters, Corcoran, & Anafarta, 2005). Attachment styles are divided into secure attachment (feelings of trust and safety), anxious-resistant insecure attachment (feelings of distress), anxious-avoidant insecure attachment (showing little emotion), and disorganized or disoriented insecure attachment (feelings of tension). As children grow, these attachment styles, as the result of their infancy, develop further and can change.

But attachment theory isn't just about how we develop as adults due to our upbringing. It also includes how adults relate to one another, especially in romantic relationships.

Adult attachment theory is based on the observation that adults in romantic relationships behave similarly in interactions to those between a child and a caregiver (Hazan & Shaver, 1987). In adult attachment theory, there are also four categories: secure, anxious-preoccupied, dismissive-avoidant, and fearful-avoidant, which correlate, respectively, with the four styles observed in children.

Depending on how an adult is oriented and how attachment styles interact interpersonally, relationships can be affected in a variety of ways. Relationship satisfaction, duration of relationships, and relationship dynamics – such as affect regulation, support, intimacy, and jealousy – can all be affected by adult attachment styles (Asendorpf & Wilpers, 2000; Collins & Freeney, 2004).

Women with eating disorders often have insecure attachment styles (Tasca, Ritchie, & Balfour, 2011; Zachrisson & Skåderud, 2010). In a 2006 study by Elgin and Pritchard, for instance, "[s]ecure attachment scores were significantly negatively correlated with body dissatisfaction" (p. 25). As such, it's possible that this experience has an effect on how women with eating disorders, and specifically anorexia nervosa, relate to their partners intimately.

Of course, hearing all of this can land in an uncomfortable way. It can seem as if the research is saying, "Women with anorexia are unfeeling and have no emotional depth; therefore, their relationships are doomed never to be satisfying."

But it's important to note that what the research is *really* telling us is that, as women with anorexia, we may be more likely to avoid intimacy – and that if we want to incorporate more emotional closeness into our lives, we can. We only first need to recognize how we contribute to our relationships.

It was this conversation about intimacy that brought me to wonder more about sensuality and skin hunger. In reading this research, I felt like we were getting so close to understanding something really interesting about the population in question, but no one was actually engaging it.

I wanted to dig in. I wanted to ask more nuanced questions about touch – ones that allowed for sexual and sensual touch to exist separately, though relatedly. I wanted to understand, if women with anorexia nervosa are less likely to desire sexual contact, but have complicated feelings about physical intimacy overall, what are their thoughts, exactly, on their experiences with sensual touch?

And this brings us to our last circle – the one that I spent years of my life trying to figure out.

REFERENCES

Advocates for Youth. (2018). *An explanation of the circles of sexuality.* Retrieved from http://www.advocatesforyouth.org/for-professionals/lesson-plans professionals/200

Aristotle. (2012). Nicomachean ethics. In R. C. Bartlett & S. D. Collins (Eds. & Trans.), *Aristotle's Nicomachean Ethics.* Chicago, IL: University of Chicago Press. (Original work published 350 BCE)

Asendorpf, J. B., & Wilpers, S. (2000). Attachment security and available support: Closely linked relationship qualities. *Journal of Social and Personal Relationships, 17*(1), 115–138.

Blackstock, C. (2011). The emergence of the breath of life theory. *Journal of Social Work Values and Ethics*, 8(1).

Bowlby, J. (1969). *Attachment and loss: Volume 1.* New York, NY: Basic Books.

Brockmeyer, T., Holtforth, M. G., Bents, H., Kämmerer, A., Herzog, W., & Friedrich, H. (2013). Interpersonal motives in anorexia nervosa: The fear of losing one's autonomy. *Journal of Clinical Psychology, 69*(3), 278–289.

Buhrmester, D., & Furman, W. (1987). The development of companionship and intimacy. *Child Development, 58*(4), 1101–1113.

Collins, N. L., & Freeney, B. C. (2004). An attachment theory perspective on closeness and intimacy. In D. J. Mashek & A. Aron (Eds.), *Handbook of closeness and intimacy* (pp. 163–188). Mahwah, NJ: Lawrence Erlbaum Associates.

Elgin, J., & Pritchard, M. (2006). Adult attachment and disordered eating in undergraduate men and women. *Journal of College Student Psychotherapy, 21*(2), 25–40.

Ghizzani, A., & Montomoli, M. (2000). Anorexia nervosa and sexuality in women: A review. *Journal of Sex Education and Therapy, 25*(1), 80–88.

Hazan, C., & Shaver, P. (1987). Romantic love conceptualized as an attachment process. *Journal of Personality and Social Psychology, 52*(3), 511–524.

Jourard, S. M. (1971). *Self-disclosure: An experimental analysis of the transparent self.* New York, NY: Wiley-Interscience.

Maslow, A. H. (1954). *Motivation and personality.* New York, NY: Harper.

Maslow, A. H. (1943). A theory of human motivation. *Psychological Review, 50*(4), 370–396. Retrieved from http://psychclassics.yorku.ca/Maslow/motivation.htm

Newton, M., Boblin, S., Brown, B., & Ciliska, D. (2005). "An engagement-distancing flux": Bringing a voice to experiences with romantic relationships for women with anorexia nervosa. *European Eating Disorders Review, 13*(5), 317–329.

Newton, M., Boblin, S., Brown, B., & Ciliska, D. (2006). Understanding intimacy for women with anorexia nervosa: A phenomenological approach. *European Eating Disorders Review, 14*(1), 43–53.

Tasca, G.A, Ritchie, K., & Balfour, L. (2011). Implications of attachment theory and research for the assessment and treatment of eating disorders. *Psychotherapy, 48*(3), 249–259.

Waters, E., Corcoran, D., & Anafarta, M. (2005). Attachment, other relationships, and the theory that all good things go together. *Human Development, 48*(1/2), 80–84.

Zachrisson, H. D., & Skåderud, F. (2010). Feelings of insecurity: Review of attachment and eating disorders. *European Eating Disorders Review, 18*, 97–106.

Sensuality

Chapter 8

What came up for me – hit me over the head, really – while researching women with anorexia nervosa and their experiences with sexuality was how little attention researchers paid to aspects of touch that were outside of a cisheteronormative definition of sex.

Most research that I read operationalized "sex" as penetrative sex between a cisgender man (penis) and cisgender woman (vagina), which is harmful (and unrepresentative) in and of itself. But researchers also tended not to conceptualize touch as broader and more far-reaching than explicitly sexual activity.

We know that women with anorexia tend to be averse to sex, I thought to myself, *but what do they feel about sensual touch? Do they like massage? Holding hands? Cuddling?*

I felt like the pursuit of this information would be an appropriate follow-up. And yet, it was rarely, if ever, explored.

And that was the moment that I changed my dissertation topic. Because I realized that as a sex researcher with a more nuanced understanding of sexuality, I could add depth to this conversation that was missing.

This chapter, then, is the longest in the book, as it encapsulates the totality of what new information I discovered in my academic journey. While what came before was mostly a cursory review of sexuality in women with anorexia nervosa as a whole, this chapter delves more deeply into the topic of touch to offer a foundational understanding of a phenomenon we've chiefly been ignoring in both research and practice: sensuality.

So what *is* sensuality anyway?

Sensuality is defined by Advocates for Youth (2018, para. 2) as "awareness and feeling about your own body and other people's bodies, especially the body of a sexual partner." Sensuality, in its simplest definition, is about how you feel in your body and how you share physical closeness with other people.

Sensuality can refer to the stimulation of any of the five senses. The sound of a crackling fire is a sensual experience. The feeling of squinting in the sun's glorious glow is a sensual experience. The smell of blueberry muffins baking in the morning is a sensual experience.

This showed up as important in my own research, as one theme that emerged from interviews with my participants was that of limited sensory awareness: They tended to have little to no memory of how their bodies interacted with their environments, especially during their eating disorder.

"I don't know that I really felt a lot of sensual experiences [during my eating disorder]," explained Talia. "In some ways...I felt not fully there." This experience of feeling not entirely present in their environments was common. Rachel elaborated on why this might be: "Being in my body has largely been uncomfortable, and I often try to sort of ignore...anything that has to do with it, [such as] any sensations I'm feeling in my body."

But the word *sensuality* is most often used colloquially to describe physical touch and tactile sensations – our experiences with being hugged, cuddled, or caressed – which explains why sensuality is often confused or conflated with sexuality, making the two sometimes difficult to differentiate between.

But they're different. If this book has taught you anything, I hope it's that many different ideas are encompassed by the word *sexuality* – sensuality included.

Helpfully, according to the Asexual Visibility and Education Network (2015), "Sensual acts are distinguished from sexual acts only by the people engaged with them...The purpose of the acts vary, as they can be an action of affection or for the purpose of sexual arousal" (para. 12).

That is, what *you* consider sexual versus sensual might not be what *I* consider sexual versus sensual. I might view a hug as an affectionate, platonic gesture; you may find hugs inherently sexually stimulating. How we interpret touch is individual – and it is also contextual. Maybe in some situations, a hug feels sexual, while in other situations, it feels friendly.

Regardless of how you interpret it, sensuality is a deeply important human experience. Touch has long been noted to be integral to psychological health, as well as a fundamental method of human interaction (Farber, 2000). "Touch," wrote Konnikova in a 2015 *New Yorker* article, "is the first of the senses to develop in the human infant, and it remains perhaps the most emotionally central throughout our lives" (para. 5).

Touch involves a wide variety of sensual experiences ruled by the somatosensory system. In regard specifically to tactile sensation, this includes negative feelings, like itches and pains, as well as positive ones, like stretches and caresses. These many sensations, which bodies are experiencing and regulating constantly, "flow from the evolved nature of our skin, nerves, and brains" in a complex biological system (Linden, 2015, p. 208). In this process, information is obtained from nerves, which travels through the spinal cord and into the parietal lobe of the cerebral cortex, where the information is processed in the primary somatosensory area of the brain.

Each nerve receptor galvanizes a different part of the brain, informing us whether we're feeling pain or pleasure, and how to react emotionally to that sensation. The nervous system interprets and responds to tactile stimuli in a variety of ways, which also vary person to person. This, for example, partially explains why some people may prefer light, medium, or deep pressure during a massage or, even more simply, are more content in colder, warmer, or more moderate climates.

However, what seems to remain mostly similar across differences is that touch plays a role in the social, emotional, physical, and cognitive health and development of all people.

And, of course, it does – it's related to our survival.

TOUCH AND HUMAN DEVELOPMENT

Oxytocin – a hormone that's involved in, among other processes, interpersonal bonding, reproduction and orgasm, and childbirth and feeding – is regularly produced by the hypothalamus, a region of the brain that's part of the limbic system. And the presence of oxytocin can generate trust, generosity, empathy, and bonding between people (Cardoso, Ellenbeogen, Sarravalle, & Linnen, 2013; Zak, Stanton, & Ahmadi, 2007). As such, it's been associated with both romantic attachment in adults and parental bonding with infants through its ability to reduce feelings of fear and anxiety in the presence of caretakers and loved ones (Bick & Dozier, 2010; Marazziti et al., 2006).

Oxytocin is what flows through our bodies and makes us feel safe and comfortable when we're being held by someone we trust. It's the warm, fuzzy feelings that accompany an embrace.

In short, oxytocin is a deeply important hormonal experience that is "with us throughout our lives" and plays a role in some of the deepest bonds that we, as humans, can experience (Moberg, 2003, p. 63).

And because oxytocin can be stimulated through sensual touch – whether massaging a baby or cuddling with a partner – it's sometimes assumed that sharing sensual experiences, then, creates, and is evident of, social benefits. That is, "if we experience friendly or loving caresses, it's safe to assume that we have a strong social network" – and not the kind that you can find online (Konnikova, 2015, para. 7).

In fact, in his 1998 book, *Grooming, Gossip, and the Evolution of Language*, Robin Dunbar made a connection between how people interact with one another and how primates groom one another: The frequency with which primates engage in grooming behaviors is a steady representation for the size and coherence of their social groups. Similarly, the experience of touch in our lives, as people, indicates high levels of closeness in our relationships.

Whoa. Hey, cousins.

Social interactions don't necessarily need touch in order to be satisfying and effective; rather, the inclusion of touch can add emotional and cognitive benefits. Research has shown that even short spurts of sensual interaction can enhance physical growth in both preterm and full-term infants (Leni, 2011; Underdown, Barlow, & Stewart-Brown, 2010). It can also improve emotional, cognitive, and physical health in adults (Field, 2001). Sensual touch has the power to affect blood pressure, heart rate, and cortisol levels, as well as stimulate positive emotions, making it effective in improving not only many physical ailments, but many psychological ones as well.

But sensuality poses some interesting challenges for women with anorexia nervosa, potentially starting from birth.

Literature on children's psychological development suggests that receiving touch from a caregiver plays a significant role in body image formation (Montagu, 1971). Freud (1923) noted that psychoneurosis is rooted in early childhood development, specifically in regard to babies' and children's interpersonal (including sensual) relationships with caregivers.

Later, Winnicott (1965) confirmed and elaborated upon this theory, remarking how mental illnesses may be related to lapses in infant development, such as the development of insecure attachment, which, as we discussed in the last chapter, is common in women with anorexia.

Touch plays a role in healthy childhood development partly in how it creates a sense of safety and comfort within family and other social systems. But moreover, touch allows young children to start to recognize the self versus outside objects – to distinguish themselves from their environments – as well as to recognize themselves as they are, which is key in the development of body image (Kuchenhoff, 1998).

In healthy development, body image evolves "into a cohesive, distinct, accurate, and consistently evocative image of one's body" and "must evolve accurately as one's physical body matures, and be integrated in the development of the psychological self" (Krueger, 2002, p. 14).

If one's body image is disturbed in childhood – for instance, through a lack of nurturing touch – then they may grow to experience more body image disturbance as they get older.

BODY IMAGE

The term *body image* was coined by Schilder (1935) to describe a person's perceptions of the aesthetics and attractiveness of one's own body: "the picture of our own body which we form in our mind, that is to say, the way in which the body appears to ourselves" (p. 11), and how we assume it to appear to others.

According to the National Eating Disorders Association (2015), body image includes what one believes about one's own appearance, how one feels about one's body, how one senses and controls one's body's movements, and can be positive or negative.

It's important to note, though, that the current definitions of *body image* within relevant fields can be limiting in how they often take a very personal, psychological perspective. Body image is also sociocultural; the effects of body oppression can have deep and lasting effects on one's body image.

In her 2018 book *The Body Is Not an Apology*, Sonya Renee Taylor explains, "Gross inequality and disenfranchisement across social experiences, poor public-health outcomes, and unjust legislation are systemic representations of centuries of infusing body shame into every sector of public and private life" (p. 50). Taylor goes so far as to write, "It is an act of terrorism against our bodies to perpetuate body shame and to support body-based oppression. I call this 'body terrorism'" (p. 53).

Indeed, the violence wielded against marginalized people at the site of their bodies must be taken into account when discussing body image as an overarching concept. It's no wonder that my own multiply marginalized participants – particularly those who were fat, trans, disabled, and/or of color – frequently named their struggles with body image as connected to overlapping oppressions.

While positive body image marks one's ability to see a "clear, true perception" of one's shape, experiencing "various parts of [one's] body as they really are" (National Eating Disorders Association, 2015, para. 3), negative body image refers to the opposite experience. Negative body image can be defined as "distorted perception" of one's body, possibly associated with feelings of shame, self-consciousness, anxiety, discomfort, or awkwardness (para. 2), which can potentially negatively impact a person's overall self-esteem and psychological wellness.

Negative body image has been shown to be a more common experience among women than it is among men (Ålgars et al., 2009; Frederick, Forbes, Grigorian, & Jarcho, 2007). And women with eating disorders especially are more likely than both unaffected women and other psychiatric populations to experience negative body image (Mangweth-Matzek, Rupp, Hausmann, Kemmler, & Biebl, 2007). Based on diagnostic criteria (American Psychiatric Association, 2013), negative body image itself often fuels anorexic symptomology.

In order to be diagnosed with anorexia nervosa, for example, one must experience "[d]isturbance in the way in which one's body weight or shape is experienced, undue influence of body weight or shape on self-evaluation, or persistent lack of recognition of the seriousness of the current low body weight," tying anorexia and body image disturbance together (American Psychiatric Association, 2013, p. 339). It's important to note, though, that while this point is useful within this conversation, the assumption of "low body weight" in people with anorexia nervosa is harmful (and also incorrect) because it leaves both fat and quote-unquote "normative" weight people out of the realm of anorexia diagnosis (OSFED notwithstanding) altogether.

Unsurprisingly, the participants in my research study expressed high levels of bodily dissatisfaction. Body image was consistently named as largely negative in childhood, with puberty and adolescence standing out as major turning points toward dissatisfaction; body image was extremely negative during their eating disorders; and they tended to find that negative body image thoughts were still present in recovery, despite behavior change.

"I've never felt completely…at home in my body," Eleana said. And Vivian noted, "I've always been self-conscious about myself."

Participants described their negative body image as so severe that they often fantasize about being able to separate from their corporeal form. "You could give me a zipper," Sarika said, "and I would unzip myself from the skin." Adra described the same phenomenon as "want[ing]…to be just a floating brain." And Cali explained that she has a "recurring daydream of just cutting myself open and dissecting out all of the fat."

Negative body image can be a precursor to eventual eating disorder development, the former being experienced before (on average, four years prior to) the development of eating disorder behaviors (Mangweth-Matzek et al., 2007). It can also be an obstacle in the maintenance of recovery efforts (Bardone-Cone et al., 2010). This means that negative body image is experienced long after the eating disorder behaviors have dissipated, creating a slew of ongoing issues in psychosocial functioning in people otherwise considered to be recovered from their eating disorders.

In my own study, 14 of my 20 participants considered themselves in recovery, and 10 of those 14 noted that their negative body image thoughts remain. Sarika noted of her eating disorder, "It's just always there, no matter what…You can always look over your shoulder, and it feels like it's just there in the room with you always."

The ways in which this negative body image impacts sexuality are varied, but they are most certainly prevalent.

In women, negative body image can lead to complications in all domains of sexual functioning and satisfaction (La Rocque & Cioe, 2011; Woertman & van den Brink, 2012). Read that again: *Negative body image can lead to complications in all domains of sexual functioning and satisfaction.* Holy shit.

Contrarily, positive body image can have a positive effect on sexual functioning and satisfaction in women, including in assertiveness, esteem, and drive (Erbil, 2011; Weaver & Byers, 2006). One 2000 study by Ackard, Kearney-Cooke, and Peterson found that, compared to women with positive perceptions of their bodies, those who experience bodily dissatisfaction reported, among other factors, less frequent sex and orgasm achievement. In fact, a 2015 *Cosmopolitan* survey also noted that 32% of women report inability to orgasm because they are, in part, "too...focused on how [they] look" (block 3).

That same 2000 study by Ackard et al. also found that women with negative body image experience less comfort initiating sexual activity, undressing in front of their partner, having sex with the lights on, and exploring new sexual activities, whereas women with positive body image reported "greater confidence in their ability to give their partner sexual pleasure" (p. 425).

A 2011 study by La Rocque and Cioe found that undergraduates with more negative body image were more likely to avoid sexual activity, which was mediated by sexual esteem, sexual satisfaction, and sexual desire. This implies that while negative body image may not directly correspond to sexual avoidance on its own, multiple related factors may lead the former to the latter.

For example, a 2013 study by Lemer, Blodgett Salafia, and Benson investigated the relationship between sexual attitudes and sexual activity in college women, with special attention paid to the potential role of body image as a mediating factor. While the researchers didn't find a clear mediation involving body image, they *did* find that more positive body image was associated with more liberal sexual attitudes, which was directly linked to more frequent sexual activity.

The potential relationship between body image and sexual activity is thought to be related mostly to the fact that "women satisfied with their body image [are] less self-conscious, [place] less importance on physical attractiveness, [are] more satisfied with their ability to form and maintain relationships, and [are] more satisfied overall with self" (Ackard et al., 2000, p. 425).

But researchers admit that while "[t]he relation between overall self satisfaction and sexual behaviors is most likely complex," still, "body image [does] play a significant role in predicting" certain sexual behaviors and attitudes (Ackard et al., 2000, p. 426).

But other connections between body image and sexual or romantic relationships can be made, too: Not only might body image affect relationships, but relationships may also affect body image, potentially creating a cycle of dissatisfaction.

A 2005 study by Sheets and Ajmere that surveyed 554 undergraduates found that over 30% of their participants in exclusive relationships had been told by a partner either to gain or to lose weight, the latter applying more frequently to women. Those participants were also found to have lower satisfaction in their relationships than the control group. And in a 2004 study by Juda, Campbell, and Crawford of relationships and women with subclinical eating disorders, it was found that participants who received low levels of support from their partners also reported an increase in diet symptomology.

This suggests that relationship health could have an impact on body image, potential weight concerns, and even eating disorders.

But here's the thing: Body image isn't only associated with how one feels *about* one's body. It's also about how one feels *in* one's body. Therefore, positive or negative body image can affect a *variety* of body perceptions.

How you perceive your body to *appear* is only one aspect of body image. How your body perceives itself in space as well as how it registers tactile sensations are others.

BODY PERCEPTION

Mindfulness is the ability to pay attention to something – in this case, the physical sensations of one's body within an environment – "in a particular way: on purpose, in the present moment, and non-judgmentally" (Kabat-Zinn, 2005, p. 4). It's the ability to be consciously aware of what's happening in the body in the present moment and acknowledging and accepting the associated feelings and thoughts that arise.

But for women with anorexia nervosa, this isn't always an easy task: Dissociation from one's physical environment is often used as an attempt to escape the physical sensations of being in their bodies.

"My body felt numb [during my eating disorder]," Talia explained. "I never had a sense of 'Oh, I'm tired' or 'I need to stop' or 'I need to slow down' or even 'I'm hungry' or 'I'm thirsty' or anything. It felt like those things didn't exist anymore."

"I wasn't actually conscious of what was going on in my body," Gina said. Cali called this experience in her body, simply, "a discomfort of being."

Participants in my study went so far as to describe a separation in their understanding of the self (or mind) and their bodies – as if their bodies didn't actually belong to them, that they were entities separate from themselves.

Rachel explained, "My body just doesn't belong to me...When I think about my body, I don't think about it as my own. I feel like...I am separate from my body." Similarly, Maia described, "I felt like [my body] wasn't me. I would have to look in the mirror and reassure myself it was me."

Of course, to someone who has never experienced this phenomenon, hearing these descriptions can sound a bit like a psychological thriller. But the experience of not being able to connect to your body is a common one for people with anorexia.

Anorexia nervosa is associated with a functional deficit of the right hemisphere of the brain, which controls various aspects of our understandings of our bodies (Grunwald et al., 2001). This may explain the experience of *multiple* body image disturbances in people affected by anorexia nervosa, as this lack of functionality can affect a multitude of somatosensory components of body representations, including the perception of touch, pressure, pain, temperature, and vibration, as well as body position and movement (Spitoni et al., 2015).

This may create a situation where people with anorexia perceive *several* stimuli differently than those unaffected – not just how they see themselves.

A 2014 review by Gaudio, Brooks, and Riva of the neuropsychological literature of non-visual sensory inputs as experienced by women with anorexia nervosa found consistent impairment in tactile (touch) and proprioceptive (position and movement) aspects of body perception.

For example, one 2011 study found that people with anorexia nervosa are more likely to overestimate distances between objects or stimuli on the body (Keizer et al., 2011). The higher their level of body dissatisfaction, the more likely participants were to inaccurately judge the mental image of their bodies, thereby overestimating the distance between stimuli being applied to their bodies. That is, if they imagined their bodies to be larger than they were, they estimated objects on their bodies to be further apart than they were. Later, a 2012 study found that people with anorexia nervosa are less likely to correctly judge the metric properties of tactile stimuli on their bodies (Keizer, Smeets, Dijkerman, van Elburg, & Postma, 2012). In this study, the researchers found that, especially when placed on the abdomen, objects would be misjudged in size by the participants.

Similarly, a 2015 study found that the brain potentially perceives touch differently based on the subject's beliefs about their own body size (Spitoni et al., 2015). Researchers reported that people with anorexia judge horizontal stimuli (tactile sensation applied along the body's width) as "significantly wider" than the same stimuli used on the body's vertical axis, which means that their brains processed touch differently, based on how big they perceived each axis to be (p. 181).

Gaudio, Brooks, and Riva (2014) summarized this issue thusly: People with anorexia have an "altered capacity…in processing and integration of bodily signals," and their "body parts are experienced as dissociated from their holistic and perceptive dimensions" (p. 1).

Traditional therapy has been shown to be ineffective in treating the specific issue of somatosensory perception (Ben-Tovim et al., 2001; Fernández-Aranda, Dahme, & Meermann, 1999). But there is hope: Some research has shown that, potentially, stimulation treatment can increase activity in the right hemisphere, thereby improving body image (Grunwald & Weiss, 2005).

In particular, the use of massage, when added to standard-of-care treatment for anorexia, has been shown to have a positive effect on both the physiological and psychological effects of the disorder. This is thought to be because massage can have an effect on anxiety, mood symptoms, negative body image, and even the biochemical abnormalities associated with eating disorders (Field et al., 1998).

For example, a 2001 study found that after five weeks, a treatment group of people with anorexia nervosa receiving massage in addition to standard care scored lower on the Eating Disorder Inventory than did those not receiving massage in addition to standard care (Hart et al., 2001).

While traditional psychotherapies may remain at the forefront of treatment, the addition of adjunctive therapies, such as massage, could enhance the treatment and recovery process.

SKIN HUNGER

I once had a partner who, for the life of him, could never remember the phrase *skin hunger.* "I'm hungry for your skin," he would tell me when he craved a hug. And I found myself constantly explaining that that sounded horrifying.

Skin hunger is not, in fact, the making of a horror film. The phrase simply refers to the extent to which a person desires sensual activity, similar to how the phrase *sex drive* describes one's desire for sex.

Advocates for Youth (2018) defines skin hunger as "[t]he need to be touched and held by others in loving, caring ways" (para. 5). They explain that skin hunger represents the need for healthy, nurturing human touch, and it doesn't need to be explicitly sexual. Activities that satiate skin hunger can include, among other behaviors, hugging, cuddling, sharing a bed to sleep in with someone, and holding hands. Skin hunger can describe anything from the need for infants to be nurtured through touch by their caregivers to young people expressing non-sexual physical intimacy with their peers to adults in sexual and/or romantic relationships who show love and care through sensual touch.

Because touch is a human need, our bodies cue us when we're not getting enough of it – similar to how we feel tired when we need sleep, thirsty when we need water, or hungry when we need food. This cue for seeking out nurturing touch, which, in abundance, can often make us feel lonely, is an experience of skin hunger. It's something that we experience throughout our lives and, like sex drive, varies in degree person-to-person and situation-to-situation.

For example, I have two cats. Halley, my sweet, senior cat, spends most of the day asleep in my bed. If and when he wants to be pet, he will find me – and meow loudly in my direction until I touch him. Astra, my baby black cat, however, needs to be in my lap all the time. As soon as I sit down, she will crawl onto my legs, curl up, and start purring. Halley has moderate skin hunger; Astra has high skin hunger.

Skin hunger, I think, is interesting because it describes a desire for touch that isn't satisfied by or encompassed within explicit sexuality. It's very obviously different, once you have it laid out for you, but isn't something we tend to acknowledge.

In reading piles and piles of articles on women with anorexia and their lack of sex drive, I was practically screaming, "Well, what about skin hunger?" Because specific data on how this population experiences this phenomenon is lacking, that feels like a pretty significant gap to me.

But there *are* related studies that provide insight into how skin hunger is situated within the experience of anorexia. In 1995, for instance, two studies came out of the University of Michigan that shined a light on the relationship between women with eating disorders and their experiences with touch. One found a correlational relationship between a woman's "current desire to get more tactile nurturance," which could be referred to as skin hunger, and her drive for thinness

(Gupta & Schork, 1995, p. 185). This suggests that women who crave more sensual touch in their lives may be more likely to also exhibit eating disorder symptoms, creating a potential connection between the two.

The other 1995 study found that touch deprivation scores for women with eating disorders were higher than for unaffected women, not only in their childhood, but also in their current, adult lives (Gupta, Gupta, Schork, & Watteel, 1995). That is, not only did these women express a wish to have received more sensual touch as children, but they also were suffering from a lack of satisfaction of skin hunger in their current relationships, romantic or otherwise.

These findings suggest that "touch deprivation may play a role in body image pathologies" (p. 459), but also that there may be a relationship between current levels of skin hunger and body image disturbance in women with anorexia.

Also, as previously discussed, in 2005 and 2006, Newton, Boblin, Brown, and Ciliska published two related phenomenological studies about how women with anorexia nervosa experience intimacy.

In the analysis of the data for these studies, the authors used a broad definition for *intimacy*. But because that definition included physical touch, some important ideas came out of these studies that apply to women with anorexia and their relationship to sensuality and skin hunger.

The women who participated in these interviews consistently expressed a lack of sexual intimacy with their romantic partners, "attributed to a lack of sexual desire and poor body image," and noted how that affects the relationship as a whole (Newton et al., 2006, p. 48). The impact of anorexia in women is that sexual intimacy is less desirous than for unaffected populations; however, some women in this study expressed that they would continue to engage in sexual activity for their partner's benefit, even though this experience was emotionally painful for them; those whose relationships lacked a sexual component expressed "the importance of its return" (Newton et al., 2005, p. 322), mostly insofar as how it affected relationship satisfaction experienced by the partner.

While participants expressed being less interested in explicitly sexual activity, though, Newton et al.'s 2005 study noted that participants expressed a need for emotional connection. This was, potentially, mitigated by participants differentiating between sexual and sensual activities: "For participants without sexual engagement, the importance of non-sexual activity" – defined here as activities such as hugging and cuddling – "was emphasized as a means of physically connecting" (p. 322).

This suggests that even women with anorexia who don't desire sexual interaction still feel a pull toward sensual touch. This is significant because it implies a need for or interest in sensual activity and a sense of skin hunger, even if an interest in sex has dissipated.

Even participants who expressed displeasure in being sexual with their partners in order to satisfy their needs did "describe pleasure from, and interest in, non-sexual aspects to experience physical closeness" again (p. 322).

But the purposeful parsing out of sensual touch from sexual touch, as a way to gauge the difference between skin hunger and sex drive, had never directly been engaged.

Thus, in my dissertation research, I set out to explore how women with anorexia nervosa make meaning of their own experiences with sensuality and skin hunger. I wanted to know not only what their experiences were, but also how they interpreted those experiences. By engaging in semi-structured interviews with 20 women of diverse identities, I discovered 21 themes in how this population talks about sensuality.

Many of those themes – such as limited sensory awareness, negative body image, and trust and autonomy – I've discussed throughout this book already. Here, I want to focus on the five themes specific to sensual touch.

SENSUAL (NON-)DESIRE

In setting out to engage in this study, I wanted to be sure of a few things: (1) that I separated sexual and sensual desire, (2) that I represented a lack of desire as normal, and (3) that participants were able to define *sexual* and *sensual desire* for themselves. As such, these conversations allowed for a lot of interpretation – both by the participants and by me, as the researcher.

I considered an experience thematic if a significant number (approximately one-quarter) of participants discussed it *or* if fewer participants (at least three) discussed it, but with gusto.

The following explores the five themes that came up in my study insofar as how participants discussed their experiences with sensual (non-)desire.

Touch Enjoyable Only with Trusted People

Approximately three-quarters of my participants named that touch is important to them or that they feel relatively neutral toward touch. "I really like physical contact," Maia said, for example. Or, as Vivian explained it, "I'm always craving touch."

Those with particularly high skin hunger expressed this need more emphatically. For instance, Gina exclaimed, "It's like I'm a cuddle whore. I fucking need them." And Farah explained, "My whole life, I have been skin hungry...I don't think I'll ever get tired of holding hands. I don't think I'll ever get tired of having our thighs touch."

Being given the opportunity to define sensual activity on their own terms, some examples that participants named as enjoyable were having their hair stroked, petting animals, engaging in eye contact, sleeping next to people, feeling someone's breath in their ear, holding children, and (I love this one!) having hearts pressed together.

However, despite the warm fuzzies that this list may have given you, participants also made it very clear that their need for touch is nuanced: Only people who they trusted were allowed to touch them. "I've always been a really touchy person, but only with certain people. Unless I'm comfortable with someone and I like them, then they absolutely cannot touch me," Kaylee explained.

For many of the women I interviewed, this meant romantic partners only. For others, very close friends and family were included. They tended to draw the line at acquaintances. "We have to be friends," Paris said, "and, like, I would say close friends."

When being touched by people who they didn't know well or didn't trust, the experience was noted to be upsetting or violating, as will be discussed in more detail later. Inari explained, "I feel like it's riskier if I don't know somebody well." And Eleana admitted, "It kind of immediately puts me on my guard."

That said, participants who enjoyed and/or especially craved touch with trusted people described these experiences as calming, comforting, soothing, joyful, happy, connecting, and healing.

Some even noted that engaging in touch with others has helped them learn to relate to their bodies in different ways, accelerating their recovery processes. "Physical contact with another [person] is one of the most healing things that we can experience," Maia said. And Eleana explained, "With an eating disorder, it's like you're being so…mean to your body that it's really good to have somebody else be nice to it." She went on, "It would just feel so nice to be reminded of what it feels like to have a physical interaction with your body that isn't harmful."

Touch Uncomfortable or Unwanted

Although far fewer participants – approximately one-quarter – noted having incredibly negative reactions to touch, those who felt this way were very strong in their emotional responses.

Participants described being touched as inducing panic and anxiety, as being presumptuous and violating. "I don't like to be touched," Maia said. "I feel trapped."

Olivia explained that touch, which she referred to as "precarious," beyond what she's comfortable with "feels like my skin is crawling." And Rachel went as far as to name that she avoids forming intimate bonds with people, both romantically and platonically, just to avoid touch.

For many of these women, personal space was a particularly important value. They expressed that they felt very strongly about their right to their own personal space and that they don't appreciate that space being breeched.

Paris described themselves as "hyperaware of people's bodies in proximity to" their own. Siobhan said, "Ever since I was a kid...I understood what boundaries are...My bubble, your bubble. You stay in [yours]; I'll stay in mine." And Cali noted, "I didn't like having another body with my body."

Lin described this feeling thusly: "If I walk down the street and someone sort of bumps into me, I feel like I have to erase it off. It's like somebody else's energy rubbing against you."

Despite this strong individual desire to have personal space respected, six participants named that there's an implied social expectation to engage in touch in order to show care toward or comfort with other people. For example, hugging people that one has not seen in a long time and shaking hands with someone that one just met are generally accepted social norms that can make some people incredibly uncomfortable.

"It's this kind of intimacy that...confirms, represents something," Inari said. Paris explained, "I know that the physical sensation of being touched is not that pleasant. But I understand, like, the importance of what it's associated with and what it means." They went on, "Honestly, if it weren't so socially significant [to engage in touch], then I probably wouldn't."

Similarly, another expectation that participants expressed as uncomfortable was that which is implied through sexual advances. For some participants, engaging in sensual touch would be comfortable, if only they didn't fear that the other party – men in particular – wanted to move that touch toward sexual activity.

Winnie explained:

If [I'm engaging in sensual touch] with somebody who might be expecting some kind of sexual experience, it's far more likely to provoke anxiety or a spiral of thoughts where it becomes uncomfortable: 'Oh my God, what am I going to be expected to do now?'

Inari said, "Even though I find [sensual touch] pleasurable, I also find it alarming. Because I feel like it's going down a dangerous path…It doesn't end with [sensual touch] with guys." She went on, "When I get to that point [when sensual touch turns sexual], I hate myself so intensely…I mean, it is serious, like, I-want-to-destroy-myself hatred."

Eating Disorder Behaviors as Expressions of Sensuality

While only three participants explicitly noted that behaviors directly associated with their eating disorders were sensual for them, it felt jarring enough a concept to include. One participant even went so far as to say that they were some of the most sensual experiences that they've ever had.

Body checking, according to the National Eating Disorders Association (2018), is "obsessive, intrusive thoughts and behaviors about body shape and size that can involve repeatedly checking appearance in the mirror, checking the size and shape of certain body parts, and/or asking others whether they look fat" (para. 13). These behaviors are, essentially, harmful ways for those with eating disorders to check the state of their bodies.

Because these common behaviors often involve touching, or otherwise sensually engaging with one's body, some participants mentioned these experiences as sensual for them. Some specific examples included touching protruding bones, engaging in exercise, grabbing fat, and measuring oneself (in inches or pounds). Eleana said, "[I would be] pinching at what was basically skin and being like, 'Look at all this fat,' and…feeling…certain parts on my body where I could feel my bones."

Participants described engaging in these activities as comforting, affirming, and even ecstasy-inducing. "When I was sick, I definitely did a lot of [body checking]," Jacinta said. She further noted that the very feeling of hunger from having not eaten was sensual for her: "I enjoy the feeling of feeling hungry. It's a distinct feeling."

Farah explained:

That was more thrilling to me [than touch from others], to be able to touch my pelvic bone and to feel it then…I loved that. That brought me so much comfort, and it was so soothing to me to be able to feel it – almost like a 'You're doing it; you're starving yourself,' like a weird affirmation.

Many of these examples feel specific to the experience of being underweight (or at the very least, thin) during one's eating disorder, as those were the experiences of the participants sharing their body checking as sensual. However, body checking behaviors can be practiced – and experienced as sensual – by anyone, regardless of size.

Thwarted Interest in Touch during Eating Disorder

Similar to how participants explained their experiences with sex drive, eight named that they were either less interested in touch during their eating disorder or are finding themselves more interested in touch now that they're in recovery.

"When restricting, the craving for touch just completely goes away," Rachel said. "And when I'm not doing so, that craving is more present."

Participants described feeling crushed, dirty, and tainted when people would touch them during the eating disorder; they also noted that the isolation induced by their eating disorder may have been related to their lack of comfort with physical contact.

"I'm more disconnected from my body [during my eating disorder]," Rachel said. "I tend to be more isolative as well… Isolating myself from other people makes touch more alien to me."

Siobhan explained, "I did not want to be touched [during my eating disorder]…because I was, in my mindset, ugly, and I needed to change." She continued, "People would just come up and hug me, and I would feel like…someone was crushing me inside…because I didn't like how my body felt."

In fact, four participants poignantly named that experiences with touch tend to be especially difficult when they're engaging in eating disorder behavior because of a fear that people can sense their body composition when touching them. "Definitely I would be self-conscious if someone was touching me," Maia said.

"It was just always a way that people could tell whether I had gained or lost weight," Olivia said. And Jacinta explained that being touched during her eating disorder made her "aware of my body and the squish."

Some participants worried that this was a purposeful act: loved ones trying to gauge their health status. Others believed that the worry was more in their own minds than in others'. "There [are] always a few suspect people," Eleana explained. "Like, 'I'm doing this to see how much weight you've lost.'"

Similarly, Sarika said, "I felt [like] if I let someone [touch me]...they would...find out, if they didn't know. Or if they already knew...they would break my [commitment to restricting], and I would somehow fall into a trap of eating."

Importantly, though, four participants expressed having *more* interest in touch during their eating disorder, namely because they needed to be reassured and comforted during this incredibly painful experience.

"When things are emotionally rough, I want to be held," Farah said. Maia explained, "I was...a lot more insecure and constantly wanting reassurance [during my eating disorder], so...I think physical contact kind of gave that to me. 'Someone cares about me. They're holding me.'"

Refusing Touch as Self-Punishment during Eating Disorder

The last common theme that emerged in discussing how participants thought about touch during their eating disorder is the idea that physical affection, especially insofar as it represents love and desirability, is something that they didn't deserve.

They would express craving touch, but not allowing themselves to engage in it – or wanting to be desired, but then pushing away those who desired them: "I wanted it, but I refused to let myself have it," Sarika said.

Similarly, Gina said, "I want touch, but once it presents its offer to me, I feel like I can't have it." She explained, "I felt like I needed to punish myself for what I was...doing."

Overall, in these conversations, participants tended to describe their feelings about sensual touch similarly to those about sexual touch, but with more enthusiasm or willingness toward sensual touch – which made this research feel important and enriching to me. Here is this population who we know is avoidant of sex, but for whom we never considered the nuance of sensual touch, telling me that *yes*, sensual touch is okay under certain circumstances.

It feels small. But for people whose sexuality has been problematized and scrutinized, this complexity can be enlightening and normalizing.

Sensuality is, indeed, its own special consideration – and we never would have known that without taking a fine-tooth comb to the concept of sexuality, breaking it down into parts.

REFERENCES

Ackard, D. M., Kearney-Cooke, A., & Peterson, C. B. (2000). Effect of body image and self image on women's sexual behaviors. *International Journal of Eating Disorders, 28*(4), 422–429.

Advocates for Youth. (2018). *An explanation of the circles of sexuality.* Retrieved from http://www.advocatesforyouth.org/for-professionals/lesson-plans professionals/200

Ålgars, M., Santtila, P., Varjonene, M., Witting, K., Johansson, A., Jerb, P., & Sandnabba, N. (2009). The adult body: How age, gender, and body mass index are related to body image. *Journal of Aging and Health, 21*(8), 1112–1132.

American Psychiatric Association. (2013). *Diagnostic and statistical manual of mental disorders* (5th ed.). Washington, DC: American Psychiatric Association.

Asexual Visibility and Education Network. (2015). *Attraction.* Retrieved from http://www.asexuality.org/wiki/index.php?title=Attraction

Bardone-Cone, A. M., Harney, M. B., Maldonado, C. R., Lawson, M. A., Robinson, D. P., Smith, R., & Tosh, A. (2010). Defining recovery from an eating disorder: Conceptualization, validation, and examination of psychosocial functioning and psychiatric comorbidity. *Behaviour Research and Therapy, 48*(3), 194–202.

Ben-Tovim, D. I., Walker, K., Gilchrist, P., Freeman, R., Kalucy, R., & Esterman, A. (2001). Outcome in patients with eating disorders: A 5-year study. *Lancet, 357*(9264), 1254–1257.

Bick, J., & Dozier, M. (2010). Mothers' and children's concentrations of oxytocin following close, physical interactions with biological and non-biological children. *Developmental Psychology, 52*(1), 100–107.

Cardoso, C., Ellenbogen, M. A., Sarravalle, L., & Linnen, A. (2013). Stress-induced negative mood moderates the relation between oxytocin administration and trust: Evidence for the tend-and-befriend response to stress? *Psychoneuroendocrinology, 38*(11), 2800–2804.

Cosmopolitan. (2015). [Infographic illustration of the results of Cosmopolitan's female orgasm survey March 16, 2015]. *Oooohhhh!: Cosmo's Female Orgasm Survey.* Retrieved from http://www.cosmopolitan.com/sex-love/news/a37812/cosmo-orgasm-survey/

Dunbar, R. (1998). *Grooming, gossip, and the evolution of language.* Cambridge, MA: Harvard University Press.

Erbil, N. (2011). The relationships between sexual function, body image, and body mass index among women. *Sexuality & Disability, 31*(1), 63–70.

Farber, S. K. (2000). *When the body is the target: Self-harm, pain, and traumatic attachments.* Lanham, MD: Rowman & Littlefield.

Fernández-Aranda, F., Dahme, B., & Meermann, R. (1999). Body image in eating disorders and analysis of its relevance: A preliminary study. *Journal of Psychosomatic Research, 47*(5), 419–428.

Field, T. (2001). *Touch.* Cambridge, MA: Massachusetts Institute of Technology.

Field, T., Schanberg, S., Kuhn, C., Field, T., Henteleff, T., Mueller, C., … Burman, I. (1998). Bulimic adolescents benefit from massage therapy. *Adolescence, 33*(131), 556.

Frederick, D. A., Forbes, G. B., Grigorian, K. E., & Jarcho, J. M. (2007). The UCLA body project I: Gender and ethnic differences in self-objectification and body satisfaction among 2,206 undergraduates. *Sex Roles, 57*(6/7), 317–327.

Freud, S. (1990). The ego and the id. In J. Strachey (Ed. & Trans.), *The ego and the id.* New York: W.W. Norton & Company. (Original work published in 1923)

Gaudio, A., Brooks, S. J., & Riva, G. (2014). Nonvisual multisensory impairment of body perception in anorexia nervosa: A systematic review of neuropsychological studies. *PLoS One, 9*(10), e110087.

Grunwald, M., Ettrich, C., Assmann, B., Dahne, A., Krause, W., Busse, F., & Gertz, H. J. (2001). Deficits in haptic perception and right parietal theta power changes in patients with anorexia nervosa before and after weight gain. *International Journal of Eating Disorders, 29*(4), 417–428.

Grunwald, M., & Weiss, T. (2005). Inducing sensory stimulation in treatment of anorexia nervosa. *Quarterly Journal of Medicine, 98*(5), 379–384.

Gupta, M. A., Gupta, A. K., Schork, N. J., & Watteel, G. N. (1995). Perceived touch deprivation and body image: Some observations among eating disordered and non-clinical subjects. *Journal of Psychosomatic Research, 39*(4), 459–464.

Gupta, M. A., & Schork, N. J. (1995). Touch deprivation has an adverse effect on body image: Some preliminary observations. *International Journal of Eating Disorders, 17*(2), 185–189.

Hart, S., Field, T., Hernandez-Reif, M., Nearing, G., Shaw, S., Schanberg, S., & Kuhn, C. (2001). Anorexia nervosa symptoms are reduced by massage therapy. *The Journal of Treatment and Prevention, 9*(4), 217–228.

Juda, M. N., Campbell, L., & Crawford, C. (2004). Dieting symptomatology in women and perceptions of social support: An evolutionary approach. *Evolution and Human Behavior, 25*(3), 200–208.

Kabat-Zinn, J. (2005). *Wherever you go, there you are: Mindfulness meditation in everyday life* (2nd ed.). New York, NY: Hyperion.

Keizer, A., Smeets, M. A. M., Dijkerman, H. C., van den Hout, M., Klugkist, I., van Elburg, A., & Postma, A. (2011). Tactile body image disturbance in anorexia nervosa. *Psychiatry Research, 190*(1), 115–120.

Keizer, A., Smeets, M. A. M., Dijkerman, H. C., van Elburg, A., & Postma, A. (2012). Aberrant somatosensory perception in anorexia nervosa. *Psychiatry Research, 200*(2/3), 530–537.

Konnikova, M. (2015). The power of touch. *The New Yorker.* Retrieved from http://www.newyorker.com/science/maria-konnikova/power-touch

Krueger, D. W. (2002). *Integrating body self and psychological self: Creating a new story in psychoanalysis and psychotherapy.* New York, NY: Routledge.

Kuchenhoff, J. (1998). The body and ego boundaries: A case study on psychoanalytic therapy with psychosomatic patients. *Psychoanalytic Inquiry, 18*(3), 368–382.

La Rocque, C. L., & Cioe, J. (2011). An evaluation of the relationship between body image and sexual avoidance. *Journal of Sex Research, 48*(4), 397–408.

Lemer, J. L., Blodgett Salafia, E. H., & Benson, K. E. (2013). The relationship between college women's sexual attitudes and sexual activity: The mediating role of body image. *International Journal of Sexual Health, 25*(2), 104–114.

Leni, E. (2011). Gentle touch and infant massage: Means to development and growth, support to child-parents interaction in premature and low birth weight newborns. *Children's Nurses: Italian Journal of Pediatric Nursing Science, 3*(4), 114–117.

Linden, D. J. (2015). *Touch: The science of hand, heart, and mind.* New York, NY: Penguin.

Mangweth-Matzek, B., Rupp, C. I., Hausmann, A., Kemmler, G., & Biebl, W. (2007). Menarche, puberty, and first sexual activities in eating-disordered patients as compared with a psychiatric and a nonpsychiatric control group. *International Journal of Eating Disorders, 40*(8), 705–710.

Marazziti, D., Dell'Osso, B., Baroni, S., Mangai, F., Catena, M., Rucci, P.,...Dell'Osso, L. (2006). A relationship between oxytocin and anxiety of romantic attachment. *Clinical Practice and Epidemiology in Mental Health, 2*:28.

Moberg, K. U. (2003). *The oxytocin factor: Tapping the hormone of calm, love, and healing.* (R. W. Francis, Trans). Cambridge, MA: Da Capo Press. (Original work published 2000)

Montagu, A. (1971). *Touching: The human significant of skin.* New York, NY: Harper & Row.

National Eating Disorders Association. (2015). *What is body image?* Retrieved from https://www.nationaleatingdisorders.org/what-body-image

National Eating Disorders Association. (2018). *Glossary.* Retrieved from https://www.nationaleatingdisorders.org/learn/glossary

Newton, M., Boblin, S., Brown, B., & Ciliska, D. (2005). "An engagement-distancing flux": Bringing a voice to experiences with romantic relationships for women with anorexia nervosa. *European Eating Disorders Review, 13*(5), 317–329.

Newton, M., Boblin, S., Brown, B., & Ciliska, D. (2006). Understanding intimacy for women with anorexia nervosa: A phenomenological approach. *European Eating Disorders Review, 14*(1), 43–53.

Schilder, P. (1935/1950). *The image and appearance of the human body: Studies in the constructive energies of the psyche.* Abingdon, UK: Routledge.

Sheets, V., & Ajmere, K. (2005). Are romantic partners a source of college students' weight concern? *Eating Behaviour, 6*(1), 1–9.

Spitoni, G. F., Serino, A., Cotugno, A., Mancini, F., Antonucci, G., & Pizzamiglio, L. (2015). The two dimensions of the body representation in women suffering from anorexia nervosa. *Psychiatry Research, 230*(2), 181–188.

Taylor, S. R. (2018). *The body is not an apology: The power of radical self-love.* Oakland, CA: Berrett-Koehler Publishers, Inc.

Underdown, A., Barlow, J., & Stewart-Brown, S. (2010). Tactile stimulation in physically healthy infants: Results of a systematic review. *Journal of Reproductive and Infant Psychology, 28*(1), 11–29.

Weaver, A. D., & Byers, E. S. (2006). The relationships among body image, body mass index, exercise, and sexual functioning in heterosexual women. *Psychology of Women Quarterly, 30*(4), 333–339.

Winnicott, D. W. (1965). *The maturational process and the facilitating environment.* New York, NY: International Universities Press.

Woertman, L., & van den Brink, F. (2012). Body image and female sexual functioning and behavior: A review. *Journal of Sex Research, 49*(2/3), 184–211.

Zak, P. J., Stanton, A. A., & Ahmadi, S. (2007). Oxytocin increases generosity in humans. *PLoS One, 2*(11), e1128.

Where Do We Go from Here?

Chapter 9

If we're not going to *do* anything moving forward, then what's the point?

Research is useful for what it elucidates in and of itself. But it's also useful in how it brings to light what we don't know – or aren't doing enough of.

There are a million different suggestions that I could offer you based on the years of research that I've done on this topic. Here, I've divided my suggestions into three overarching categories: those for eating disorder practitioners, for advocates, and for researchers. I imagine, if you've got this book in your metaphorical hand, you fall into one of these categories.

Here is what I would like to see us doing now.

EATING DISORDER PRACTITIONERS

In the services that many practitioners who work with eating disorder clients provide, there is often already a base-level understanding of how eating disorders and sexuality can interact. This sets a clear foundation for the value that various healthcare providers place on sexuality as a cause and an effect of eating disorder experiences.

Here, I'm simply making recommendations specifically from a sexological perspective – that is, how practitioners can continue and expand upon their support, given what we know specifically about sexuality.

Recognize Sexuality as a Broad Topic

Sexuality is a vast topic; there are various ways in which sexuality affects human experience. Sexuality is more than just behavior and reproduction. It's more than what you do, who you're into, and how your body works.

Sexuality includes the intimacy of emotional risk-taking and sharing vulnerability. It includes aspects of identity, such as gender, orientation, and performance. It includes what people think and know about sexuality, from both values- and information-based perspectives. It includes sexualization and objectification, fantasy and sensuality. And so much more.

Sexuality is a complicated web of identities and experiences, interacting to form individual histories and expressions. If you've gotten anything out of this book, I hope that it's this understanding.

Without a foundational understanding that sexuality is complex and all-encompassing, it can be difficult to address the issues within it. However, outside of the study of sexuality, little attention is paid to how broad and far-reaching sexuality can be. As such, training in sexuality from a sexological perspective could be helpful to eating disorder practitioners in order to gauge a fuller picture of how clients experience sexuality.

The work being done with clients – in therapy, medicine, nutrition, and other sciences – can be enriched by a clearer, more nuanced understanding of sexuality. Exploring opportunities to work with consultants and training leaders for professional development in the science of sexuality is the first recommendation, as this knowledge can lay the groundwork for deeper work at sexuality's intersection with eating disorders.

Understand the Relationship between Trauma and Eating Disorders

A continued effort to understand the causes and effects between histories of violence and eating disorders is necessary.

Within therapeutic environments, broadening this exploration beyond sexual assault can be helpful: It's necessary to understand how other abuses (physical, emotional, and so on) may have similar effects, as that can provide more clues to understanding how eating disorders develop, how to treat them, and how to work with clients in healing their relationships to sexuality.

When sexuality is understood as something broader than the behavior that often defines it, it becomes clearer how various aspects of a person's life can interrupt their ability to connect to themselves and others sexually.

Learn a Thing or Two about Sensate Focus

For those who are specifically working with women with anorexia nervosa (or any population, really) on the issues with which they are struggling within the physical realm of sexuality, an exploration of sensate focus may be helpful.

Sensate focus is a practice coined and created by Masters and Johnson (1970) that involves slowly (re)introducing sensual touch into a person's life and/or relationship with partner(s) in a deliberate manner. It encourages exploration of and connection to tactile sensations, especially to promote mindfulness of one's own experience.

This practice is often guided by a sex therapist. As such, referring clients to sex therapy if touch is an issue for them, and if the practitioner has no training in sex therapy, is a possible solution. A sex therapist can guide clients through the various stages of sensate focus – moving from non-sexual touch, to the inclusion of common erogenous zones, eventually to the inclusion of genital touch and intercourse – to help develop comfort with and appreciation for sensual touch gradually.

Note that for some, self-exploration may be an important first step before moving into partnered activities.

Continue to Center Mindfulness

Continuing to center mindfulness and grounding activities in recovery, especially in terms of healing and treating experiences of dissociation, is helpful.

This may be true in general for women with eating disorders, given the disruption of mind-body connection, but it could potentially be especially true for those who are struggling with various aspects of sexuality.

Practitioners are given an opportunity to assist in the recovery process of those with eating disorders. And those clients deserve to work with the most knowledgeable and compassionate people. Understanding sexuality from a nuanced perspective can help practitioners provide the best care for their clients.

EATING DISORDER AND SEXUALITY ADVOCATES

Advocacy around both sexuality and eating disorders is an effort necessary to engage in from a social justice standpoint, especially insofar as how these experiences interact. Engaging in this research only increased my own personal awareness of how important this work is.

In conversations with the 20 participants who took part in my study, the hundreds of people who I have addressed in writing and speaking about these issues, and family and friends who have taken an interest in my research, I have come to understand just how desperately people are craving information on this topic.

As such, here are recommendations for advocacy efforts.

Spread the Word about the Vastness of Sexuality

As I discussed previously in the recommendations for practitioners, a broader understanding of sexuality is of utmost importance.

Working – particularly as sex educators, therapists, and researchers – to disseminate accessible information about the vastness of sexuality should be foundational. Only from a place of acknowledging how various aspects of sexuality interact can more specific issues be tackled. Sexuality affects people's lives in myriad ways; as advocates, we must address that.

Within my research specifically, this need was especially evident insofar as how people separate their understanding of sexual and sensual desire. Parsing out the latter from the former, allowing and encouraging people to explore them separately, if interconnectedly, seemed to be a powerful permission, especially for women who experience them differently. This allows people the opportunity to deepen their conceptualization of their own sexuality and to gain a better understanding of how touch presents itself in their lives.

Talking about touch from a standpoint that is not explicitly sexual may not inherently feel critical or radical. However, teaching people how to explore sexuality in ways they hadn't considered – indeed, in ways that may be more comfortable and validating for them – can be life-changing.

Understand How Sexuality Presents Differently for People with Eating Disorders

Within this same vein of accessibility of information, helping women with anorexia nervosa – as well as other eating disorders – understand that their experiences are common can help disrupt this population's feelings of abnormality.

Many women in my study expressed concern about how "weird" or "strange" they were. Unbeknownst to them, they were actually expressing experiences similar to other participants and reflective of prior research.

Given the opportunity to redefine normality in sexual behavior could save women years of grief and shame. That sexual experiences vary and that normality is non-existent is an important part of the advocacy conversation.

Normalize Asexuality

The normalization of the asexuality spectrum is necessary, including in terms of how women with anorexia nervosa experience touch.

That I couldn't find any published research that explored the intersection of asexuality and eating disorders, despite decades of research exploring a lack of sex drive in women with anorexia nervosa, is astounding.

Although only a few participants in my own study actively identified as asexual, those who did found power and validation in the label and community.

Discussions around sexuality must include asexuality as a valid and common expression, giving language to an experience with which many may be struggling, especially in a sexually charged culture.

Consent Education Must Include All Kinds of Touch

The conversation around consent, which is increasingly popular and gaining more nuance, must include all kinds of touch.

It should be made clear that touching another person's body is only appropriate with non-coerced permission. This includes hugging, holding or shaking hands, and even pats on the back that feel congratulatory and soft caresses meant to express concern.

No one should be put in a position to feel uncomfortable or violated by touch; as advocates, it's necessary to explore this further and to set the foundation for consent at seemingly innocuous touch – not just explicitly sexual interactions.

Advocacy can go so far in offering public awareness and personal affirmation. As such, it's the duty of those who wish to advocate on the behalf of people with eating disorders to be knowledgeable about sexuality (and vice versa) and to prioritize lesser-publicized issues.

FURTHER RESEARCH

The focus of eating disorder research currently leans toward finding neurobiological causes (and potentially, cures) for eating disorders. But since eating disorders have such large, everlasting effects on those affected, more attention must be paid to various changes in people's experiences due to their eating disorders. This includes sexuality.

Similarly, while sexuality research includes body image and beauty standards, the nuance of eating disorders is often missing. There is a lot of untapped information waiting to be discovered at this intersection.

Here are recommendations for moving forward in the realm of research.

Take My Research and Run with It

A larger-scale exploration of the themes found in my study could allow for a better sense of generalizability.

Having the opportunity to interview only 20 participants leads to a small sample size and not enough information necessarily to make grand statements about the phenomena herein.

Further studying this phenomenon within this population with a larger, nationally representative sample can expand upon these results. Even better, perhaps eventually moving this research to a large-scale quantitative study, after the creation of an instrument that was shown to gauge these experiences reliably and validly, could do even more to suggest generalizability.

Do More to Explore Sensuality and Skin Hunger

My research focused specifically on women and anorexia nervosa; however, there are more genders than women, and there are more eating disorders than anorexia.

Exploring the topics of sensuality and skin hunger in people of all genders with all eating disorders could be informative in understanding how anorexia nervosa, bulimia nervosa, and binge eating disorder interact with these phenomena differently.

Specifically, while research explores how women with anorexia and bulimia experience sexual functioning and sex drive, both the newness of binge eating disorder as a diagnosable eating disorder and the recent changes to diagnostic criteria for anorexia and bulimia mean that some of this research may be in need of updating.

Furthermore, the lack of inclusion of people of other genders leads to incomplete research. After gathering this foundation, comparing experiences with sex drive to skin hunger would be illuminating.

Go Ahead and Disclose

Beyond topics for future inquiry, however, is also the question of methodology.

I have experienced within professional eating disorder spaces a strong pull toward avoiding self-disclosure. This led to a personal struggle when designing and carrying out my research study. The question of whether or not I should self-disclose my own eating disorder history was difficult to work through.

However, in prioritizing Patricia Hill Collins' "ethic of care" (1989), by which "personal expressiveness, emotions, and empathy" are considered "central to the knowledge validation process" (p. 766), I came to the conclusion that self-disclosure was appropriate. My first few interviews were conducted in a manner by which I held myself back. It wasn't until I gave myself permission to be comfortable in the interviews, including being authentic about my own experience, that the interviews flowed more easily and richly.

In their anonymous post-interview surveys, participants even named this honesty as helpful to them within the interviews: "Having someone who was coming from a place of understanding made it a very comfortable experience," one participant wrote. Another explained, "It was...nice to talk to a fellow eating disorder survivor because I don't get [that opportunity] often."

Methodologically, self-disclosure should be reconsidered as a potential *benefit* to research, rather than an assumed disadvantage or breach of professionalism.

Despite issues for marginalized populations within the spheres of academia and research institutions, research can provide a powerful opportunity to better understand – and then solve – problems.

This group deserves attention from the scientific community – and moreover, a nuanced approach to understanding their experiences.

Luckily, there are people who are excited to do that work – and I know that some of you are included in that group.

REFERENCES

Collins, P. H. (1989). The social construction of black feminist thought. *Signs, 14*(4), 745–773.

Masters, W. H., & Johnson, V. E. (1970). *Human sexual inadequacy.* New York, NY: Bantam Books.

Where Do We Go from Here?

Afterword

Studying the intersection of eating disorders and sexuality has often been a lonely, exhausting process. From the frustration of having to fight for sexuality as a worthwhile conversation in the eating disorder world, to the confusion of using the acronym "ED" in a room full of sexuality peers who immediately assume *erectile dysfunction*, to the emotionally harrowing process of interviewing 20 women about a topic that can still be triggering for me, this has not always been easy. And it hasn't always been fun.

What has been most meaningful for me throughout, though, has been the excitement with which my project has been met from the folks who matter most: eating disorder sufferers and survivors who have never been given a space to talk about their sexuality, even sexuality professionals who have never had a chance to discuss their eating disorders. In conference presentations, social media posts, and one-on-one conversations, I am continually met with people's desire for this information – their need to have cobwebbed parts of them validated. It always leaves me with a sense of awe.

I wrote this book for them – for you. I wrote it because this information is hard to find, made even more impossible if you don't have access to academic language, let alone a university library system. I wrote it because our relationships to our bodies – and the trauma they bear – are so complex and delicate, and we are rarely given opportunity to unpack that. I wrote it because I know there are people out there who wonder if their eating disorder is related to their sexuality, but don't have anyone to ask. And I wrote it for the people who care about them, whether platonically, romantically, or professionally.

Together, we must demand that this conversation continues. We must bring the topic up, even in seemingly inappropriate places. We have to fight to make sure that sexuality spaces honor eating disorders, that the eating disorder field takes sexuality seriously. As educators, researchers, service providers, and advocates, we must validate the experiences within these pages and create opportunity for others to explore their own histories. We have to be brave in the face of conflict.

And most of all, as we consider how our bodies exist in biological, psychological, and sociopolitical spaces, we must learn to trust them.

Index